CW00822026

The Handbook of Jungian F
with Children and Adolesce.

The Handbook of Jungian Play Therapy with Children and Adolescents

Eric J. Green

With a Foreword by John Allan

JOHNS HOPKINS UNIVERSITY PRESS   BALTIMORE

Note to the reader: The discussions and procedures herein are intended to acquaint readers with some of the techniques of Jungian Play Therapy that can be helpful in providing emotional and psychological care for children. It is intended to provide information to help children *in general,* and not to help any specific child. The views expressed are not necessarily the views of the author or of the publisher. This book is not meant to substitute for medical or psychological treatment, and treatment should not be based solely on its contents.

© 2014 Johns Hopkins University Press
All rights reserved. Published 2014
Printed in the United States of America on acid-free paper
9 8 7 6 5 4 3 2 1

Johns Hopkins University Press
2715 North Charles Street
Baltimore, Maryland 21218-4363
www.press.jhu.edu

Library of Congress Cataloging-in-Publication Data
Green, Eric J., author.
   The handbook of Jungian play therapy with children and adolescents /
Eric J. Green ; with a foreword by John Allan.
      p. ;   cm.
   Includes bibliographical references and index.
   ISBN 978-1-4214-1510-9 (pbk. : alk. paper) — ISBN 1-4214-1510-0 (pbk. : alk. paper)
— ISBN 978-1-4214-1511-6 (electronic) — ISBN 1-4214-1511-9 (electronic)
   I. Title.
   [DNLM: 1. Play Therapy—methods. 2. Adolescent. 3. Child. 4. Jungian Theory.
5. Professional-Patient Relations. WS 350.4]
   RJ505.P6
   616.89'1653—dc23   2014004980

A catalog record for this book is available from the British Library.

Special discounts are available for bulk purchases of this book. For more information, please contact Special Sales at 410-516-6936 or specialsales@press.jhu.edu.

Johns Hopkins University Press uses environmentally friendly book materials, including recycled text paper that is composed of at least 30 percent post-consumer waste, whenever possible.

He was my North, my South, my East and West,
My working week and my Sunday rest.
—W. H. Auden

This one's for you, Paul, my great mentor.
It was the BEST time of my life.

Contents

Foreword

Ten years ago I was lecturing at the University of North Texas in Denton, and a young man approached me at the end of the workshop, saying he had read much of what I had published, found it inspirational, and would like to offer his services to me as a researcher and cowriter. I thanked him for his comments and generous offer and said that right now I did not need any research or writing help. I added that I thought the most important thing was for him to do his own research, on play therapy with children and families, and to write up and publish his findings. I am very pleased to say that this young man was Dr. Eric Green and that this book, *The Handbook of Jungian Play Therapy with Children and Adolescents,* is the fruit of the combination of his playful energy and hard work over the past ten years.

Dr. Green has written a very important book—the first of its kind to specifically address Jungian Play Therapy with children and families. In part I, the theory section of the book, Dr. Green shows a deep understanding of Jung's major constructs and how they both elucidate our understanding of the psyche and facilitate treatment. He provides a clear definition of terms and a discussion of four broad archetypal categories, and includes such areas as the shadow, anima-animus, the self, the ego-self axis, death-into-rebirth, and symbol amplification. He quotes from Jung and addresses issues of the transference-counter-transference and the importance of the therapist "maintaining an analytical attitude" throughout treatment. He pays attention to issues of "time and space": the classroom, school, or community center represents "ordinary time," but the playroom is the "sealed vessel," the "vas" (the container), the place for "sacred time," where the psychological transformation occurs. There are important rituals (or awareness) for entering and exiting this sacred space ("the *temenos*") with the child and family members. Dr. Green shows how, through play and fantasy enactment in the playroom, emotions are expressed physically and/or symbolically, wounds are healed, and the child and family are freed of trauma, neglect, or developmental blocks to move forward and to grow.

What is impressive about this book is the sheer range of children, adolescents, families, and situations that Dr. Green has worked with. This book is truly a "Handbook of Jungian Play Therapy with Children and Adolescents"! His cases cover many childhood struggles and situations, including physical and sexual abuse, depression, bereavement, autism, witnessing of violence, ADHD, "daydreaming," self-injurious behavior, and children and families affected by such natural disasters as flooding, hurricanes, and tornadoes.

The book will be very useful to many students and practitioners, because Dr. Green has been trained and is experienced in a wide range of theories and techniques. He integrates these in an overall Jungian frame that makes the new learning accessible to many therapists. One clearly sees how Dr. Green considers himself part of a team of mental health workers—he consults with parents, teachers, and psychologists and articulates a treatment plan for each child and family. He uses evidence-based research findings to inform his practice. He sees the child alone in the playroom but then, when appropriate, incorporates parents and at times teachers in the room at later dates. He is not rigid or dogmatic but rather lets the child and the situation direct the flow of treatment. Dr. Green clearly enjoys children and has a very soulful practice.

The book is replete with useful symbolic activities to use with children, adolescents, and parents. As Dr. Green explains, the symbol contains emotions, and as the symbol evolves through play, so does the child's inner emotional world, and children begin to develop a rich internal life, which in turn facilitates learning, attending to schoolwork, and making friends. We see patterns in children's play, movement from chaos to struggle, and finally resolution. At this point play therapy is no longer necessary and the child terminates treatment, often with a statement like "I don't think I need to come and see you anymore."

The child's self-healing and creativity are encouraged through engagement in a variety of expressive arts techniques, including such therapist-suggested activities as coloring a mandala, sand worlds, directed and spontaneous drawings, self-portraits, journals and letter writing, guided imagery (including "My Guardian Spirit"), playing calming music tapes, and the reading of stories, myths, and fairy tales. Dr. Green selects the activities based on the psychological makeup of the child. For example, with a child who has Asperger's who spent a lot of time looking at himself in the mirror, he chose to read and discuss the Greek myth of Echo and Narcissus and then asked the child to "sand a picture from the story." As the child worked in the sand, he made a spontaneous statement: "Me and him both like mirrors." This timely intervention (the reading of the myth and the sand activity) opened up a whole new part of the child, which enabled him to disclose to Dr. Green and to change outside of the playroom with family members and other children.

In this case study and others throughout the book, Dr. Green gives many examples of his responses to and interpretations of the child's struggles. The reader becomes aware of Dr. Green's ability to empathically mirror the deeper emotions of the children and to provide the words and language to help children understand themselves and move forward into new growth. These are important counseling skills to demonstrate, so that readers are left with a new set of constructs and verbal skills for their own use. But at the same time, as shown in many of the cases, Dr. Green also models the ability of the therapist "to remain silent and to witness" the unfolding of the child's psyche without the distraction of words and interpretations.

This brings us to the difficult question of how to be a therapist, or more specifically the difference between "the role of the therapist" and "the therapist as a person," and how to straddle those two stances. Successful therapy is surely a mixture of the two. Jung described the therapeutic relationship as "an existential encounter between two people where, by the end of treatment, both client and therapist change." Like Jung, Dr. Green stresses the paradox: one should be very well trained in theory and at the same time "throw it all out of the window" and be present with the immediacy of the child and the family. The danger is that if therapists are too heavily bound by theory, they will miss seeing and hearing what the child is feeling and doing in the moment and will leave the child feeling unseen and abandoned. However, if they are not well enough trained in theory, they will not be able to develop an "analytical attitude" to understand the depth and meaning of a child's struggle.

Dr. Green shows how the therapist can take risks and act spontaneously while with families and children. For example, with one early adolescent he takes his shoes off and engages the child at the child's level, thus getting out of the child's power play, changing the expectation the child has of the adult, giving the child a new and different experience of adults, and helping the child find new solutions to old, entrenched problems.

At times Dr. Green's writing style is quite percussive and very physical. This is a good attribute, because he is both bold and embodied. The text is alive and imaginative, and it encourages therapists to be alive and creative in their work. Dr. Green "talks" to readers and encourages them to paint, draw, do sand pictures, and engage in "active imagination" themselves, before, during, and after the therapy sessions and while reading the book! He also emphasizes the importance of the therapist's own therapy and remaining in supervision (either individually or in groups) while treating children and families. This book will be useful to readers and hold their attention for many years.

John Allan, Jungian Analyst
Professor Emeritus, Counseling Psychology
Faculty of Education, University of British Columbia
Vancouver, Canada

Preface

Soul enters life from below, through the cracks, finding an opening
into life where functioning breaks down.

—Thomas Moore

———

When I was a child, my uncle Paul, a Jungian-oriented Catholic priest, used to read passages to me from the Christian Bible, Thomas
Moore, and Joseph Campbell, as well as snippets of the collected works of
Carl Jung. From a very young age, I remember looking up to my uncle and
wanting to like some of the same things he enjoyed, as he was an intellectual
and extremely cultured. Later on, he took me on many trips, infusing his
Judeo-Christian, progressive beliefs with Jung's psychology as part of our
cultural experiences. I remember having a lengthy discussion with him, at
about 13 years old, while playing *Scrabble,* about Jungian archetypes and the
collective unconscious. I wasn't quite sure what it all meant; but with consistent study and curiosity, I began to internalize the more psycho-spiritual
aspects of Jung's teachings. I took up interest in the Enneagram and the
Myers-Briggs. And I attribute this early interest in Jung and his teachings
solely to the influence of my uncle. This parlayed itself into my now lifelong
journey of studying, teaching, writing, and incorporating Jung's archetypal
psychology into clinical practice with children. It was in my very early youth
that my love affair with analytical psychology took shape and form. I am
still attracted to Jung's writings and the modern revisions from the post-
Jungians because of the emphasis on the soul and the "soul making" that occurs through reaching the depths described within Jungian psychoanalysis.

While I was completing my doctoral work, I was employed as an elementary school counselor in New Orleans, Louisiana. Having studied Jung in
my graduate school curriculum, and subsequently having attended several
educational workshops in archetypal psychology from Jungian institutes
(they are typically found in many major cities across the United States), I
created a "Color Your Mandala" self-awareness curriculum at the elementary
school where I was employed. We conducted the typical classroom guidance

lessons and from within that developmentally sensitive paradigm asked children to draw and color their mandalas (or "magic circles") based upon identifying and relating to central themes from the stories we read. Many of the children reported a decrease in anxiety while drawing the mandalas, and there was observational and qualitative data suggesting that some of the children began to cultivate a rich inner life that assisted them in making better choices in their external environment. The following is a response from a 5-year-old female: "Doing the mandalas helped me understand my mother better, and now I don't want to fight with her as much." I also used sandplay when working with children in individual sessions at my elementary school, and they found it fun, relaxing, and helpful to clear their minds and work out different scenarios to difficult problems within their sand pictures. For more information about my research during this period, please refer to my doctoral dissertation, "Elementary School Children's Perceptions of Play Therapy," which can be found by navigating to http://scholarworks.uno.edu /td/262/.

To further demonstrate the applicability to diverse clinical areas, a team of play therapists, school counselors, and I used Jungian Play Therapy techniques in south Louisiana with large numbers of displaced children following Hurricanes Katrina and Rita. Our team initially focused on Psychological First Aid; and then later, we incorporated serial drawings and sandplay to help some of the children integrate the cognitive processing of their potentially traumatic events. Our team's work was featured in the CNN television documentary *Children of the Storm*. In the summer of 2013, I was part of a team, led by Jennifer Baggerly, that provided disaster mental health services to the children and families affected by the deadly tornadoes that killed seven children at one elementary school in Moore, Oklahoma. While we provided disaster mental health–Psychological First Aid, we also integrated some of the analytical play therapy interventions mentioned in this book, including sandplay and analytical expressive art therapy interventions, such as "Dream Your Dream On" and "Color Your Mandala." We performed pre- and post-tests with the children and families, as well as administering biofeedback and deep-breathing exercises to decrease anxiety. The results of this initiative demonstrated that the interventions produced a decrease in anxiety surrounding the negative event in many of the child participants. These examples, and many more articulated later in this book, will provide the rationale and operationalization of using Jungian Play

Therapy with children in schools and communities as a potentially helpful paradigm.

For those of you who have found your way to this book, I warmly invite you to join me in the process of demystifying the erudite theory that Carl Jung conceived at the turn of the twentieth century. As a graduate student in a counseling, psychology, or social work degree program, or an elementary / middle / high school counselor, or a practitioner in private practice or for a not-for-profit organization, you may have developed an appreciation for "depth approaches" with children and may be looking for new ways to make your work with children and families even more meaningful. The central aim of writing this book is for you, the reader and child mental health practitioner, to have unfettered intellectual and emotional access to analytical theory, technique, and application, so that you may integrate these concepts and operationalize the techniques in your clinical work.

For far too long, there has been a tacit understanding, however misguided, that Jungian psychology was too complex for the typical master's-degree-level clinician to utilize, or perhaps required years of expensive training in a remote part of the world (Zurich, Switzerland). It is my argument that there is enough common sense in these techniques and applications for most master's-level clinicians to successfully begin the process of augmenting their style and clinical approaches to incorporate the analytical attitude, theoretical precepts, and practical applications outlined in this book. Anyone with a basic relationship to his internal or symbolic life, a minimum of a master's degree in a mental health field, and a mental health license, may utilize these practical techniques without years of formalized, expensive Jungian-based training and personal analysis. Dora Kalff, the woman who conceived the term *sandplay,* was a brilliant therapist, and at times her children played with Jung's children. She had no formal training in play therapy at the time when Jung asked her to study under Margaret Lowenfield, but she developed this rich technique of using sand and miniatures in a container to project one's rich, psychological interior.

Your quest to integrate analytical play therapy approaches, including sandplay and coloring mandalas, will not end after reading this book. Rather, the book may be just the beginning. I encourage you to make learning about depth approaches part of your lifelong educational journey. To ethically continue with your learning during and long after you read this book and as you utilize the ideas presented, you may want to (a) seek out professional conferences and workshops that focus on analytical designs and/or play therapy with children, (b) locate the latest books from your local library written on psychodynamic approaches and play therapy with children, (c) engage in personal counseling to work on awareness/integration of your shadow(s) and projections, (d) participate in a regular supervision group with other clinicians using play therapy and/or analytical approaches when working with children, and (e) eventually participate in more formalized, in-depth training from a Jungian framework, including becoming credentialed by the Sandplay Therapists of America as a sandplay therapist.

The book is organized in a straightforward manner so that the reader may maximize the intersubjective field dynamics between a therapist and a child client. The first chapter, on Jungian Play Therapy, will be a refresher for most master's and doctoral level clinicians, after your graduate coursework. I've included information specific to Jungian Play Therapy to fully realize the underpinnings of what makes the theory (as applied to children) helpful and practical. Instead of using one dense chapter to deconstruct some of the dizzying terms and often contradictory language we find in some of Jung's writings, I've incorporated the theoretical concepts throughout the chapters with simple explanations supplied. As part I of the book lays the foundation of knowledge, part II applies these concepts to approaches and techniques that may be used with children in elementary and middle schools, community agencies, and private practices. Part III builds upon the first two parts cumulatively to present the knowledge and skills as applied to diverse clinical populations. This section is included for the reader to hopefully make meaningful connections between her current psychotherapy practice and the applications in analytical play.

This theory, analytical play therapy, as I've conceptualized it from a post-modern Jungian perspective, accentuates the beauty in child psychotherapy in its artful nature and the inherent mystery arising from symbols maintained within that beauty. For some readers, parts of this book may make you feel like going back *home* to where many of us began this journey of becoming practitioners—recognizing the need for a balance between the art and the science of psychotherapy and the need to not polarize one or the other, because there the inevitable shadow appears. Some of you have lost your way from the original path that led you into this field in the first place, mainly to use whatever is available to ethically and effectively connect with and help children in need. You may feel that you cannot possibly keep up with the constant influx of new and often contradictory research findings that emerge every few months. Still, some of you are looking for creative mechanisms to make your clinical work meaningful and remain effective as a caring practitioner who honors the caring for the soul (yet still be accountable to insurance companies for third-party reimbursement). Whatever your reaction or impetus in reading this volume, I implore you to take this journey with me to the end. And whatever end result may come about, know that I wish you well as you seek to influence children's psyches so that they may lead emotionally rich, meaningful lives and find their own way toward the healing trajectory.

In his meta-analysis in the *American Psychologist* of February–March 2010, Jonathan Shedler stated that psychodynamic (or analytical) therapies, those approaches that include not only symptom remission (which is the primary aim of most evidence-based, behavioral approaches) but also the distinguishing feature of fostering positive psychological capacities (i.e., creating meaningful relationships, relating to symbols in one's fantasies and dreams, healing complex emotional scars from childhood to promote resilience and positive self-worth, etc.), demonstrate high effect sizes in the treatment of mental health disorders, as compared to those of cognitive behavioral therapy, or CBT. Shedler identified multiple factors specific to the psychodynamic (also "depth" or "analytical" psychology) approaches that may be anomalous to new, scientific, and primarily behavioral evidence-based treatment approaches: (a) focus on affect and expression of emotion, (b) identification of themes and recurring patterns, (c) focus on the therapy relationship, and (d) the exploration of fantasy life.

A simplistic or reductionist view would indicate that the pendulum of psychotherapeutic debate within the community of scholars often swings between the depth or humanistic approaches on the left and the manualized, evidence-based treatment approaches figuratively on the right. At the time of the writing of this book, it seems as though there is evidence to support clinicians drawing upon both systems of thought and scientific inquiry to honor the *psyche* (soul) as well as cognitive and neurobiological implications derived from evidence-informed, modernized practices. This book's primary aim is to add depth to the literature on child play psychotherapy, the pendulum swing toward the left, so to speak, while maintaining an appreciation of and a connection, however tenuous, to the evidence-informed basis of treatment and the associated treatment effect size of change. Should one want to delve more into the theory behind Jungian child psychotherapy, beyond the cursory bit contained in this book, *Inscapes* is a terrific place to start. It should also be noted that Dr. Allan's book and his subsequent writings over the past 25-plus years have *significantly* influenced the research contained within this book.

Getting back to this preface's aim, the overarching goal of Jungian Play Therapy (JPT) is activating the *individuation process* (i.e., becoming a whole, psychological individual) in childhood. The process is facilitated through a warm, empathic relationship between a trained adult and a child, in which an analytical or symbolic attitude is cultivated within a *vas,* or a container that imbues psychological safety. The goal of individuation is operationalized through the transformation of symbol—the process of the child's symbols being generated throughout therapy. Jungian play therapists observe symbol production and transformation in children throughout the clinical process. The therapist *honors* (or observes without judgment) images so that children can regulate their impulses and maintain equilibrium of energy flow between their inner and outer worlds.

The analytical attitude of the therapist permits the child to move from impulse or action to the symbolic life, where emotions and images are contained. By containing rage, therapists facilitate children's transformative process, sublimating aggression into assertiveness, which brings forth positive feelings. Through the safety of the therapeutic dyad, aggression moves into assertiveness to help children articulate, "I do not like or I am mad" instead of loathing or physically attacking toys or others. This dyad brings about healing as the child internalizes the "good enough" parental *imago* (image). The use of symbols in dreams and the therapeutic use of symbolic play enjoy a rich tradition that has occupied a central place from the beginning of child psychoanalysis. Let these prefatory comments serve as an invitation to the reader to place preconceived ideas of Jungian therapy with children aside, open your mind to the beauty of working with symbols, and allow the process of learning about this dynamic play therapy to unfold organically.

A Jungian perspective on a cure in treatment occurs when a play therapist facilitates the activation of the child's self-healing archetype. This occurs by encouraging creativity and accepting the inexplicable mystery and psychic energy associated with the unconscious symbol. Specifically, symbols tell children where they are in the therapeutic journey by pointing to the area of the unconscious that is most neglected. The Jungian therapist unconditionally accepts that position and supports the child unconditionally along the therapeutic journey. After the self-healing symbol in play appears, the therapist explores the child's inner thoughts and feelings by reconciling the meaning of the symbol, with the assistance of the child. After a successful integration occurs, termination follows (this varies with individual client needs, ranging from three months to two years).

Each chapter contains a bit of the theoretical underpinnings of analytical or depth psychology in relation to children's symbols of self-healing in play therapy. Then, the chapters provide practical techniques for clinicians to incorporate into their work. Finally, clear, easy-to-understand case studies are presented to illustrate the Jungian Play Therapy application in diverse clinical populations within elementary and middle schools, community agencies, and private practices. All of the clinical case studies presented in this book are derived from my part-time clinical practice in child and family psychotherapy over the past several years and my previous work as an elementary school counselor and as a disaster mental health responder. All information identifying the clients within the case studies has been altered and disguised to protect client confidentiality.

The Jungian perspective provided throughout this manuscript reflects some of the classic Jungian school of thought, as well as integrating post-Jungian thinking, such as archetypal psychology, as espoused by Michael Fordham and Maria Soldi and modernized by John Allan. This book emphasizes that self-healing or individuation can occur in childhood through the precondition of a nonjudgmental, caring, therapeutic dyad. This statement, for some readers, may sound similar to the therapeutic assertions made within child-centered or nondirective play therapy. At times, it has been difficult for some clinicians and theoreticians to differentiate Jungian Play Therapy from nondirective play therapy. One of the reasons for this is that Jungian Play Therapy, like many other play therapy schools of thought, utilizes some of the nondirective micro-counseling skills (such as reflecting feeling, content, setting limits) within psychotherapy with children. This premise is not dissimilar to major theoretical psychology models that have many features in common with the person-centered therapy of Carl Rogers and Virginia Axline. One of my aims in writing this book is to present a clear, concise overview of Jungian Play Therapy so that clinicians will be able to integrate practical techniques correlated to Jungian theory, a depth approach, into their existing models to enhance practice, especially the techniques that come from the complementary paradigm of nondirective play therapy. I have devoted part III of the book (almost 50% of it) to Jungian-specific applications to children, so that the reader will have a clear idea of how this modality differs and complements nondirective and other major theoretical models.

It is my hope that you will join me on the journey of reading this book and will continue the process of deepening your already meaningful mental health work with children and their families. It is my aim to make the techniques and applications outlined here comprehensible enough and easy enough for typical master's level clinicians to implement in their practice. Please feel free to visit my website (www.drericgreen.com) for colored versions of the pictures contained in this volume, as well as my contact information, should you have any comments or questions as you embrace the depth approach and continue your own clinical journey in this field with children.

Let the journey outlined in this book provide you, the reader, with guidance for your own heroic journey toward integrating Jungian or analytical play therapy competently and ethically into your current child psychotherapy practice. Developing as a Jungian play therapist takes many years of personal analysis, engagement in professional development trainings regarding symbols and shadow and archetypes (and various archetypal psychology seminars), a firm commitment to cultivating the symbolic attitude, recognizing soulfulness while honoring the spirit, and finally a consistent effort to rediscover enchantment in simple things, including nature and *beauty*—love's invisible embrace. When integrating Jungian play into your practice, remember this outline: (1) know your own foundational theory backward and forward (inside and out) and have years of practice within a variety of modalities with diverse clients; (2) identify elements of this theory that you would like to incorporate into your own by keeping a journal as you read this book, highlighting the concepts, ideas, and techniques that your clients may find useful; (3) study this book, then find the DVD *Jungian Play Therapy and Sandplay with Children,* to see the concepts and interventions applied in real scenarios with real children; (4) seek out supervision from a Jungian-oriented supervisor, mentor, or analyst in your area to provide guidance and support for you along the way; (5) engage in consistent critical reflection throughout the process (what worked, what didn't, and why?); (6) be undergoing your own personal analysis or counseling during the integration process so that you may contain the projections and be aware of your shadow; (7) document or videotape your counseling sessions with the integrative pieces so that you may watch them and self-evaluate; and (8) continue to undertake additional professional development trainings on this topic and reflect back to your own integrative practice, refining and renewing.

To prepare you for the personal and professional development that lies ahead at the heart of this book, let's start by engaging in a reflective activity. If you have a sand tray and sand miniatures nearby, consider this activity: close your eyes and do some deep breathing, centering your mind, clearing your thoughts, relaxing your body, and then open your eyes again. Just make sure it's a free and protected space so that there are no cell phones, interruptions from others, alarms, or distractions. You, the sand, the symbols, and silence will unite for the next 20–45 minutes or so. Create a sand picture, anything you'd like. There's no right or wrong way to do this. After you're done, absorb the images by noticing them. Perhaps take a picture of your sand creation. Perhaps journal about what it may mean to you if you want, or feel free to not journal or think about the meaning at all. If you do not have a sand tray, you can draw a circle on a blank white piece of paper. Create your mandala. Again, there is no right or wrong way. You may want to play peaceful, relaxing music softly in the background as you create. You can use colored pencils, buttons, glue, glitter, crayons—whatever you'd like. When you're done, consider journaling about the mandala. But you do not have to. If you do decide to reflect and share your thoughts and feelings through writing, consider the story of the mandala. Consider the title the mandala may have. Consider how this may relate to some part of you or your life as a snapshot right now in some context. After you've finished with your sand picture or mandala drawing, take a few moments to just "be." No more writing or reflecting or checklists from a book you're reading. Just sit with yourself and the images for 10–15 minutes and see what emerges. This, my friend, is the beginning of your newest heroic journey as you begin this book and integrate analytical play into your practice. But more than that, this is about integrating an experience of depth or the divine into your personality. Remember what Jung said: it is your personality alone that will decide (not the theories or techniques). At the end of the book, we will pick up from here and complete another experiential activity to provide closure for the book and the journey, and honor the new beginnings your soul has led you to.

Two editorial notes: First, all figures of children's sand and artwork are reproductions by the author of the children's original renderings during their treatment. Second, portions of the book are adapted from the author's previous publications and appear here with permission of the publishers. Chapter 4 is adapted from E. Green, The crisis of family separation following traumatic mass destruction: Jungian Play Therapy in the aftermath of hurricane Katrina, in N. B. Webb, ed., *Play therapy with children in crisis: Individual, group, and family treatment*, pp. 368–88, 3rd ed. (New York: Guilford Press, 2007). Chapters 5–8 are adaptations from the author's previously published work in the *International Journal of Play Therapy (IJPT)*; they are used with expressed permission of the Association for Play Therapy. Chapter 5 is adapted from E. J. Green, A. Myrick, & D. Crenshaw, Toward secure attachment in adolescent relational development: Advancements from sandplay and expressive play-based interventions, *IJPT*, 22 (2) (2013): 90–102; chapter 6 is adapted from E. J. Green, Re-visioning a Jungian Play Therapy approach with child sexual assault survivors, *IJPT*, 17 (2) (2008): 102–21; chapter 7 is adapted from E. J. Green, A. Drewes, & J. Kominski, The use of mandalas in Jungian Play Therapy with adolescents diagnosed with ADHD: Implications for play therapists, *IJPT*, 22 (3) (2013): 159–72; chapter 8 is adapted from E. J. Green & M. Connolly, Jungian family sandplay with bereaved children: Implications for play therapists, *IJPT*, 18 (2) (2009): 84–98. Chapter 9 is adapted from E. J. Green, The Narcissus myth, resplendent reflections, and self-healing: A contemporary Jungian perspective on counseling high-functioning Autistic children, in L. Gallo-Lopez & L. Rubin (eds.), *Play-based interventions for children and adolescents with Autism spectrum disorders*, pp. 177–92 (London: Routledge, 2012).

Acknowledgments

First, I want to humbly thank Jacqueline Wehmueller and Sara Cleary at Johns Hopkins University Press for believing in this project and seeing it through. Thank you.

Second, I want to gratefully acknowledge John Allan, who wrote the foreword. It's a distinct privilege to call you a friend and mentor. "Your spirit is shining, surrounded by love."

Third, I want to thank my closest friends and family, including Belinda and Gerry Green, Anthony Shaw, Cordell Robinson, Jana Doughty, Rev. Msgr. Paul Metrejean, Ilene Pearce, Fred Hanna (my spiritual brother!), Nichole Burgess, Joseph Northcutt, Jose Ortiz, and Daniel Schlinke.

Thanks to the colleagues who've shown consummate support: Athena Drewes, Charles Schaefer, Judi Parson, David Crenshaw, Jodi Crane, Kalpana Saxena, Kathryn Elliot, Rhonda Bryant, Sueann Kenney-Noziska (one of my favorite play therapists on this Earth!), Mistie Barnes, JoEllen Holmes, Kathy Lebby, Kim Rubenstein (for seeing the good in me, even when I won't), Mary Guindon, Pilar Hernandez-Wolfe (for "Act 2" of my career), Elizabeth Robey, Theresa Coyne Fraser, Jo Downs, Dee Preston Dillon, Cher Edwards and Linda Homeyer (for writing letters of support during tenure so I could finish this book in peace!), Linda Dench and Sandra McSwain (great champions of play in PA), Larry Epp and Duane Isava (unwavering support and dear colleagues from MD), Anne Stewart (oh how I love you so!), Gina Eustaquio and Liz Kong, Sandra Frick-Helms, Christina Koehler and Marshia Allen-Auguston (for making mentoring meaningful); and especially Eliana Gil.

John Seymour: thanks for being an external reviewer for this book and a loyal friend over the years.

Jennifer Baggerly: "Though the mountains may crumble, and the hills may come to an end; my love will not desert you. My promise shall not be broken" (Isaiah 54:10).

Ilene Pearce: my Jewish mother and eternal cheerleader. You would not let me give up on this book. Thank you for the sweetness, for it shows.

Amie Myrick: thanks for your help with formatting this project and for allowing me the privilege to collaborate with you time and time again.

JP Lilly: your contributions to Jungian Play Therapy through APT and your work with BACA have helped to keep the model alive and children safe. It's an honor to know you.

Dean Santos, Judith Nix, Provost Becker, President Brown, Brenda Robertson, and my entire UNT faculty colleagues: for allowing me the time and space to do what I love. Thanks for trusting me.

Deanne and Harry at www.SelfEsteemShop.com and Gary Yorke at www.ChildTherapyToys.com for selling my Jungian Play Therapy books and merchandise . . . thanks for your loyalty over the years!

Harriet Friedman, Rie Rogers Mitchell, and Jackie Kelly: thank you for warmly welcoming me to the Sandplay Therapists of America.

Cheryl Holcomb-McCoy, Ileana Gonzalez, and Norma Day-Vines: for inviting me back each summer to teach and form meaningful relationships with our students. Thank you for keeping this Johns Hopkins University connection alive and well over the years.

And finally, I want to extend the biggest thanks to my students. I fumble toward "ecstasy" time and time again. Thanks for granting me the privilege to learn from you more than you ever learn from me. And know that most of what I do, besides for the kids, is for you.

I JUNGIAN PLAY THERAPY

Theory

1

Identifying the Self-Healing Archetype

Childhood is the time when, terrifying or encouraging, those farseeing dreams appear before the soul of the child, shaping his whole destiny.

—Carl Jung

———

This chapter begins with a brief discussion of Jung's archetypal theory as applied to children in play psychotherapy. Jungian Play Therapy (JPT) is a dynamic, creative approach to counseling children that emphasizes symbolic meaning. Jung believed that children's psyches contain a transcendent function—an innate striving for personality integration—that occurs through symbolic identification. Clinicians may promote psychic healing in children by emphasizing the salience of the positive therapeutic dyad and facilitating the emergence of the self-healing archetype that is embedded within children's psyches. A self-healing archetype is an innate symbol that promotes healing by helping the child recognize and achieve a balanced communication between the ego and the Self. By reconciling polarities, children facilitate inner healing by resolving dichotomous feeling tones in archetypal complexes—complexes centering primarily on the struggles between good and evil, shame and pride, and condemnation and redemption. Various micro-counseling skills involved in Jungian Play Therapy are presented, including, but not limited to, interpretation and analysis.

The term *analysis,* implied from Jung's theory of analytical psychology, which is what Jungian Play Therapy (JPT) is based upon, refers to reducing complexities into firm, simpler components. In play therapy with children, analysis occurs as a therapist listens to and observes a child in his play and social interactions, to ultimately help the child come to awareness and reduce stress (Fordham, 1994a). JPT is a vibrant, creative approach to counseling children that involves the analysis of symbolic meaning (Jung, 1959), which corresponds to the existentialist and humanistic "care of the soul" (Yalom, 1995). Swiss psychiatrist Carl G. Jung (1875–1961) believed the psyche contained a *transcendent function* (an innate striving for personality integration) that occurs by producing symbols and allowing them to lead toward healing. Children's symbols, or *archetypes,* are understood from the individual perspective or phenomenological viewpoint of the child. Archetypes are bipolar feeling tones made up of (a) spiritual energy and (b) feelings associated with culturally specific images in human behavior that may appear in dreams, fantasies, and mythology, such as Earth Mother, Trickster, and Wise Old Man (Green, 2009a). In other words, the therapist does not arrogantly apply a predetermined meaning to symbols produced in the psychotherapy through dreams, sandplay, or drawings: It is up to the child to attribute her own meaning to the symbols produced. There is no right or wrong attributional basis when deciphering symbolic meanings in play psychotherapy: it is how the child makes sense of the symbols that imbues the healing.

Analytical play therapists facilitate a therapeutic environment for children to develop their own path toward self-healing by nonjudgmentally attending to children and identifying the emergence of the *self-healing archetype* that is embedded within children's psyches (Allan & Clark, 1984; Green, 2007). A self-healing archetype is an innate symbol that promotes psycho-spiritual healing by recognizing and achieving a balance between the demands of the *ego* and the *Self.* Articulated simply, the ego is the seat or faculty of reasoning (the "I" as we know it), and the Self is the ego aligned with the personality (perhaps the "soul"). The child's self-healing archetype is activated through symbols produced through the creativity and active imagination inherent in play (Allan, 1988). In other words, symbols point to the area of the child's unconscious that is most neglected. By integrating opposites, children achieve equilibrium between the burdens of the ego and the external world (e.g., home, school, peers), on one hand, and the needs of the personal unconscious (the inner world of feelings and fantasies), on the other. The activation of the archetype is accomplished as the therapist illuminates the unconscious by connecting the inner world of the child to the outer world. This is done in analytical play through the intersubjective process of cultural and archetypal contextualization. Practically speaking, this can be done simply by a therapist incorporating fairy tales into the psychotherapy so that a child may draw images from the story and by the use of symbols and sandplay (see information later in the chapter on fairy tales). Identifying the self-healing archetype in the play process, which sometimes appears as a sun in a child's drawing or a gold treasure chest in a child's sand picture, possibly indicates that the child is engaged in the self-healing trajectory and may be an indicator that therapeutic termination may not be too far off.

Jungian Play Therapy: Overview

Both Allan (1988) and Green (2007) identified JPT as a beneficial treatment modality when counseling elementary-school-aged children. Additionally, several qualitative investigations and anecdotal data obtained through case study analyses have demonstrated JPT as a beneficial therapeutic modality with young children struggling with difficult feelings and behaviors (Allan 1988; Allan & Bertoia, 1992; Allan & Brown, 1993; Allan & Clark, 1984; Green, 2006, 2007). The conceptual basis of JPT is that during children's development, either by *introjection* (internalizing beliefs of others) or *identification* (strongly relating to the values and feelings of others), feelings, thoughts, and traits of primary caretakers are acquired (or internalized), as well as any associated dysfunction or trauma(s) related to those significant primary relationships. Therefore, the practice and scope of JPT is to afford children sufficient psychological space in an emotionally protected environment or *vas* (container) so that personal development (i.e., *individuation*) materializes. Individuation characterizes a progress from psychological fragmentation toward wholeness: It is the acknowledgment and reconciliation of opposites (i.e., integrating dichotomous feelings and thoughts) within an individual (Jung, 1951). Therapists promote self-healing through the safety inherent within a nonjudgmental and accepting relationship that is not based on changing a child, but accepting the child. As mentioned previously, archetypes appear throughout the play therapy process, since they form the basis of typical activities and behaviors associated with the human existence, which are evolutionary and upon which individual development proceeds (Stevens, 2006). In JPT, archetypes represent the unconscious link between psychic events occurring within the consulting room and feeling events occurring outside the consulting room (they serve as unconscious visuals, so to speak, that link the child's inner and outer experiences).

While archetypes are discussed in more detail in chapter 2, it is important to note that there are typical archetypal themes that manifest in analytical play therapy with children that may be helpful for the reader to consider now, in this introductory chapter on JPT. These archetypal themes organize children's behaviors and affect and may be codified into four broad categories: (1) *archetypal events:* Birth, Separation from Caretakers, Initiation; (2) *archetypal figures:* Wise Old Man, Earth Mother, Trickster, Hero, Divine Child; Death; (3) *archetypal symbols:* Sun, Moon, Water, Mandala, Cross, Fish, Sea; and (4) *archetypal motifs:* Creation, Dark Night of the Soul, and Revelation (Green, 2009a).

The central premise of JPT is the salience of the child's relationship to the symbolic life, or, how children relate to the symbols they produce through dream work, drawings, fantasies, free play, puppet theater, and sandplay. From a Jungian perspective, inner development occurs when an individual acknowledges and creates symbols from dreams and fantasies and follows these symbols wherever they lead through active imagination. Moreover, Jungian therapists stay *at the feeling level* of the child when integrating the symbols of healing throughout the play process. Ego therapists sometimes want to rush in, but analytical play therapists try to remain patient observers. Jungians recognize that children must be treated in their own right as individuals (Fordham, 1994b), and not viewed merely as a symptom within a dysfunctional family system. Before moving into the symbolic phase in clinical work, therapists must build trust with children by initially accepting who they are. Once trust is formed, the child's unconscious is freed of situational anxiety and may be more likely to engage in symbol production. As children produce symbols in play therapy, Jungians indicate that they "enter the symbol"; or, put another way, the symbol de-integrates or is reduced to a conscious feeling or recognizable image for the child and can be contained. For example, if an introverted child presents with anxiety or ADHD, the therapist will witness what image surfaces with the child's neurosis by assisting the child in switching off the ego's energies and painting the image of anxiety. Jungians believe that by entering the feeling, one can change the feeling.

Therapeutic Goals

The predominant goal of JPT is activating the individuation process in children through an analytical attitude, where images are produced. Once images and elements within the unconscious are made conscious, children can better regulate their impulses by maintaining equilibrium of energy between their inner and outer worlds. Individuation is operationalized through the transformation of symbol—the process of the child's inner symbols being generated throughout therapy. Children speak through actions and metaphor in symbols, so Jungian-oriented play therapists may pay close attention to the things not talked about or enacted during a session. Everything that transpires in the playroom and right outside the playroom (e.g., as when the parents arrive with the child) is clinical data to be considered and carefully analyzed by the therapist.

A second goal in JPT is for both the child and the therapist to develop and maintain an *analytical attitude*. Fordham (1994a) describes the analytical attitude as a technique that provides conditions for children to freely express themselves while a therapist emphasizes interpretative rather than directive methods. The essential feature of the analytical attitude is that it is impartial and seeks to illuminate the child's conflicts and resolve them in the present moment. The analytical attitude of the therapist permits the child to move from impulse or action to the symbolic life, where emotions and images are contained. Therapists facilitate children's transformative process, which brings forth affective containment. For example, a child used a book she did not like as a makeshift door stopper in the playroom. While the therapist set no limits on this action, the child became even more incensed, because she wanted or expected the therapist to punish her in the same way her mother typically did when she engaged in self-expression. For context, her mother's harsh punishments were the reason she was referred to therapy by one of her teachers. The therapist noticed the dynamics and modeled the analytical attitude by taking off his shoes. The child laughed and said, "Mr. Green, what are you doing?" The therapist replied, "I never did like these shoes. My mom bought them for me at Christmas. I saw how you used the book as a door stopper to show how you don't care for it, so

I'm going to take off my shoes for the rest of the day and not wear them again." The child responded in a laughing tone of disbelief, "You need to do your own sandplay. You have problems too! Maybe I can hide the book on the bookshelf so I can't see it, if you put your shoes back on. Your socks are smelly." From this exchange, the child was able to contain her disdain for an object and sought a viable alternative in the present moment without being directly guided or manipulated into it. The therapist stayed with the symbol and metaphor of the play, which indicated that something undesirable needs to be removed to decrease anxiety. However, young children do not have the developmental or language capacity to discriminate that information, so they do things similar to what this child did and use books they don't like as door stoppers to show their discontent. This is an example of modeling the symbolic or analytical attitude and staying with a metaphor with a child to bring about change in the present moment.

Another goal of JPT is to *ground* (stabilize or reorient) children from their rage or aggression and gently help them move back to the less-symbolic, more concrete external reality. This must be done gently, as it can be jarring and disorienting to a child to go from one extreme of deep symbol work to another extreme of leaving the session and walking to fourth-period science class. In other words, children cannot engage in the headiness of symbols and then be expected to participate in most typical, structured types of activity immediately afterward. They need time to internalize the symbols and feeling tones quietly, if only for a few moments. Parents may be encouraged to leave the car radio on mute when they enter their car with the child after a play session, allowing silence to permeate for five minutes. Another practical example of grounding is when a child is directed by a play therapist to draw at the conclusion of a therapy session (Green, 2009a). The transition of drawing at the end of a play session helps a child move his rage from impulse to action. Children must be permitted to symbolically and behaviorally abreact rage within the consulting room without consternation or fear of retribution from the therapist. Furthermore, play therapists *carry* the child's aggression or rage, thereby aiding them in relieving some of the associated anxieties from the aberrant feelings. This is done by having the child draw and externalize the flood of visuals produced by the psyche in the playroom. In contrast to many Western psychotherapists' ideals, rage is not seen as something adverse in the child that needs to be remedied or "cured." Intense and conflicted emotions, along with the behaviors that stem from these emotions, are not eliminated, necessarily, so the child may conform to society. Instead, the Jungian-oriented play therapist sensitively supports children so that they may eventually come to accept themselves as unique and complete, aberrant feelings and all. This does not mean the therapist permits the child to engage in hurtful or destructive behaviors toward the therapist to provide an all-accepting platform for expression. It does mean that feelings are accepted as valid, but behaviors are modified if they involve hurting others.

Another JPT goal is for children to internalize images of the "good enough mother" and "good enough father" (Winnicott, 1971), so that they can nurture themselves or engage in self-nurturing after the course of psychotherapy ends. Play therapists, however strange this may sound, are always looking to work themselves out of a job, since that would be the point where the child and the family are able to move on and cope with life again without the outside assistance of a therapist. It is also important to note that therapists are present in the consulting room neither to meet the emotional needs of children nor to get their own needs met. The dialectic should remain in a forward-moving direction in that therapists help children become aware of difficulties or limitations so that children accept and/or resolve them at their own pace and inclination. Through self-nurturance, an internalization of a positive self-image may emerge by a child identifying with the good mother archetype or the good father archetype internalized from the caring behaviors demonstrated by the therapist. Practically, this appears in the playroom when the child voluntarily incorporates the therapist in drawings and sand pictures and free play. Jungian play therapists assist children in reconciling the meaning of the good enough mother and good enough father images activated within the playroom by the therapist by (a) asking what the symbol means to the child and by (b) asking the child to externalize the accompanying inner dialogue associated with the symbol. For example, if a 6-year-old draws variations of an eagle, which in some cultures represents parental wisdom or perceived authority, the therapist may ask questions related to the eagle to understand the child's relation to the symbol. Then the therapist may attempt to amplify (explore) the symbol by asking the child questions or making comments such as, "Let's talk about the eagle and what its purpose is in this drawing. Does the eagle live alone or with others?" "Is the eagle ever afraid or brave or both? When?" As the therapist actively dialogues with the symbols within children's drawings, their egos are provided a voice to express inner longings, desires, and hidden or unknown attributes related to internalizing a good mother or good father image.

Treatment Description

The consulting room (playroom) and the child's ritual entrance into the consulting room are akin to the symbolic ritual of initiation in that one moves from the *profane* to the *sacred*. The clinical experience of entering and resolving psychological issues within a playroom resembles cultural, tribal, and primordial forms of initiation. For example, the Oglala Sioux, a group of Native American Indians who refer to themselves as *Lakota*, participate in vision quests (Sherwood, 2007). Vision quests are spiritual initiations for those seeking to move into adulthood or higher states of consciousness. Often, the archetypal rite of initiation is constellated around difficult physical symptoms, psychological unrest, unexplainable emotional turmoil, or death of a loved one and may involve a spirited dance and/or burning herbs and lighting candles. While therapists are not expected to burn leaves or engage in vision quests every time children enter the playroom, perhaps clinicians may consider lighting a votive candle or playing relaxing music as the child arrives. This sets the scene of migrating into a serene or sacred space. The third-century alchemist Zosimos of Panopolis referred to the psychological distress before initiation begins as the *unendurable torment*. For initiation to occur, some type of *temenos* or sacred space needs to be present (e.g., in JPT, the playroom), with a human guide or shaman (e.g., the play therapist), and there must be stages of submission, disorientation, containment, and reorientation. The shaman metaphor coincides with the Jungian therapist, as both move into the patient's unconscious and wrestle with emotional demons. The vision quest is an initiation into a deeper relationship to the mystery of life, as the goal of Jungian Play Therapy is individuation, the child's path of self-discovery through a reconciliation of opposites that provides the energy for inner transformation.

The playroom, or *temenos,* should be child-friendly and developmentally appropriate. A child-friendly playroom may contain a couple of sand trays (one wet and one dry) and several hundred sand miniatures and objects depicting various feeling tones and archetypes that children can use to manipulate in the sand and create a picture. The sand miniatures are culturally inclusive, with figures from various religions, including the Star of David or the menorah from Judaism, an icon (e.g., the Virgin Mary) or crucifix from Christianity, and the Buddha statue from Buddhism. Sand minis should also include multicultural representations of individuals, including family figures of Asian, Mexican, Caucasian, African, and Indian descent.

In addition to a sand tray and miniatures, the Jungian playroom contains a puppet or playhouse, where the child may hide. This is essential for the playroom so that children may perceive a sense of emotional safety by relegating their ego to a hidden place that is impenetrable should they encounter difficult raw material while playing out themes in the playroom. Another reason to maintain a hiding place in a clinical playroom is that a child may want to relax and ease her psyche from the frenetic pace of the school day. The "hidden place" permits the child's ego to escape from the external environment temporarily and regenerate itself in its solitude. The playhouse puppets are multicultural and contain representations from various professions. Moreover, the play therapist ensures that sexist stereotypes are not reinforced in the playroom, and male and female puppets represent different professions, including doctors, firefighters, police officers, and so forth.

Within the safety of the puppet house or playhouse, a covered space where a child's ego can *hide,* the analytical therapist is able to differentiate threats to the child's ego through the projections contained within the drama. The play drama occurring inside the puppet house is viewed as an extension of the child's unconscious, where hidden conflicts are brought to the surface and given a voice within the safety of the playroom. The analytical play therapist links those projections to the child's reality by providing a voice to the child's pain. Here is an example of dialogue between "Alicia," a 9-year-old child client, and her therapist, who were engaged in puppet play within the consulting room:

> *Alicia:* This family is happy, or not. Here's the father, who's nice to everybody. But maybe not. And the little girl is happy, because her sister doesn't bother her.
>
> *Dr. Green:* It seems as though everyone in this family tries to get along. But maybe there is still a lot of pain and hurt occurring.
>
> *Alicia:* Well, sometimes, maybe the dad comes home, and he's had a bad day at work and yells, "OK, you kids need to listen to me, or I'm going to get mad. And you don't want that." (Alicia picks up the little girl figure and speaks.) "I picked up my room daddy. But I accidentally spilled my grape Kool-Aid on

the carpet." (Then Alicia returns to the father figure and speaks in a stern voice.) "Girl, you never listen. And I'm going to spank you for spilling on my white carpet. When will you learn?"

Dr. Green (staying with the metaphor): Sounds like the daughter may be upset and hurt by the mean things her dad said to her. I bet she wishes she was big like her mother is so she could make the rules and not always be told what to do.

Alicia: Yeah, she does. She's tired of always being told what to do. She wants to be the boss. She can't do anything about it 'cause she's a kid. She wants to run away sometimes.

Dr. Green: Sounds like that little girl feels helpless and gets so angry and hurt by the things her dad tells her that she doesn't know what to do with those feelings. I wonder if she sees that her dad loves her, but maybe he's sad too and needs help himself. (Therapist talks directly to little-girl figure in kitchen.) "Can you show me how you feel right now and what you can you do with those feelings?" (Green, 2009a)

In this dialogue from puppet play, the therapist stays at the feeling level of the child, which seems to be hurt and hopelessness. The therapist gives a voice to Alicia's rage by exploring the hurt within the child puppet figure, which Alicia uses as a representation of the current dilemma at home. Once Alicia's storytelling changes to be less critical and slightly hopeful, the interpretations made by the therapist change slightly to embody hope. Children often engage in this type of metaphorical play, because it is less threatening to communicate difficult feelings about caretakers they love.

Techniques

First, the play therapist and child must *surrender* the demands of the ego to micro-manage the relationship-building process. Instead, the therapist must allow the process of rapport building to organically flourish, based upon a trusting, emotionally safe (i.e., nonthreatening and caring) therapeutic alliance over time. As Stein (2007) notes, it is important for the play therapist to attend to subtle interactions in the analytical relationship while simultaneously engendering an emotional holding environment in which the child's ego feels safe to reveal itself. Typically, rapport-building begins at the very first encounter with a child. The therapist squats or matches the physical level of the child, looks the child in the eye, smiles, respects physical space and proximity, and warmly and genuinely exchanges names and welcomes the child into the room for a special playtime. The child's entrance into the playroom (or the sacred space) and the therapist's unconscious shape the progress of the nascent therapeutic dyad.

A second specific strategy is *analysis of the transference.* Transference, within a Jungian framework, as intimated earlier in this chapter, is not solely projections of the child's personal past (e.g., parent complexes) onto the therapist, but also archetypal or nonpersonal projections the child unwittingly transfers onto the therapist. The central aim of analyzing the transference is not to figure out what happened that brought the child to therapy, but how to repair what happened in the present moment through the therapeutic relationship. Unlike Freud, Jung emphasized the importance of current conflicts constellated in the transference as more important than the interpretation and analysis of the child's past infantile rage or pathology. Furthermore, when working in the transference, Jungians not only acknowledge the problems that happened in the child's past; they also acknowledge that these problems are healed in the present moment through the corrective emotional experience inherent within the therapeutic relationship (Sedgwick, 2001). Because of this commingling of the *wounded* child and the sensitivities of the therapist's personality, the transference sometimes creates a feeling of inadequacy for the therapist. For example, "Alicia" was playing in the sand tray by dumping large amounts of sand onto the floor, and his play therapist felt overwhelmed. When these types of feelings occur, typically symbolizing the emergence of the Self, the therapist must place the feelings into words. When Alicia was manipulating a mother figure in the sand picture that was responsible for the sand dumping, the therapist commented, "I wonder if the mother in that scene feels angry and overwhelmed and doesn't know what else to do except rebel?" Working from the transference, the therapist becomes aware of his and the child's feelings in play and articulates these feelings to the child's ego. In this example, the therapist attempted to solidify the language of what Alicia's ego was expressing through sandplay, "So Alicia, the mother in the sand picture is really angry, and she wants everyone around her to feel some of that pain." Within the transference, the therapist "carried" some of the child's psychological poison (Allan, 1988) and subsequently gave a voice to Alicia's hopelessness and terror. Consequently, the mother sand figure stopped dumping the sand on the floor and began scolding the children sand figures in the sandbox for making her so angry that she "throw out all our sand." Alicia moved from impulse to action here and sublimated rage into the less potent form of rage—aggression.

A third JPT strategy is *amplification of symbols*. Jungian play therapists attempt to amplify symbols contained within play, which means the therapist makes them conscious or obvious through verbal and nonverbal play interventions (De Domenico, 1994). Often, active imagination is used to help the child produce inner symbols so that the Self may lead the child toward healing. Jung's definition of a symbol implies that it in itself is not able to be portrayed; instead, a symbol is the totality whose manifestations can be observed in the joining of the psyche's elements (Fordham, 1994b). Practically, amplification involves a therapist identifying a dominant symbol in a child's drawing or sandplay and asking the child to create a new drawing or sand picture based upon the most significant struggle presented by the child in the previous play. In this activity, the child enters the symbol and often changes it, with new perspectives and ideas on old problems. So if a child draws a mandala with a bird in the middle that is killing others, perhaps the therapist may amplify the symbol by asking the child to create a new mandala and show what caused the bird to become so murderous. Affect changes only when it's externalized.

To amplify symbols in drawings or dreams, Allan (1988) suggests that the therapist use one or possibly two of the following probes with a child: (a) Do these symbols tell a story? (b) Can you tell me what is happening in this scene? (c) If you were inside this (therapist points to symbol or image), what would it be like? (d) What went on in the story before this image appeared? (e) What happens next? (f) Could you tell me what you were thinking or feeling as you drew/sanded this? (g) What does this (therapist selects a specific object or symbol) mean to you? and (h) If you could give this a title, what would it be? During the process of amplifying symbols in children's play, the play therapist provides verbal and nonverbal communications that reflect unconditional support, so that children will come to realize that happy and scary feelings are acceptable to express in the therapeutic relationship. Through making meaning of symbols and amplifying their affect, children harness the necessary ego-energies to attenuate the various assaults to the ego in a typical day at school or at home.

The final objective of JPT is for a therapist to provide interpretations to the child during play where psychological disturbances, which are the underpinnings of complex defenses (such as the *shadow*), may be reached (in other words, helping the child come to terms with the unconscious). For example, if a child is playing with a dollhouse and continues to show a doll being beheaded by a male figure because she didn't clean her room properly (this child was embarrassed at school the week before by her teacher after she wet her panties. The teacher's humiliating and dramatic comment to the child in front of her classmates was, "This is the third time you wet your pants this week. Off with your head, little girl"). The therapist then responded with an interpretation, "Seems like she's not feeling good about herself because she can't clean her room as fast and as well as her older sisters. And that mean guy there is beheading her over and over to show her punishment. It must be a terribly frightening, scary, and unsafe world to live in. Maybe the little girl can talk to her older sisters and see if anyone can help her clean her room so she doesn't have to keep getting humiliated by that mean male figure." She then smiled, stopped the beheadings, and said, "Yeah. I think that's just what she'll do." The child sought the counsel of her sisters about overcoming her anxiety, which led her to wet her pants at times. They told her that she must be brave and when she feels like she has to go to the bathroom, she should go. Now, while this information was hardly revelatory, because it came from her similar age-group siblings, whom she cherished, the message finally stuck. She had no more accidents at school again after that point.

The purpose of interpretation is to bring unconscious contents into awareness and to help the child mediate anxiety. The technique of interpretation gives the child information about his therapist's capacity to (a) hear him, (b) see him, (c) understand him, and (d) ultimately accept him. It is a key inductive technique in Jungian Play Therapy, because it provides the child the abilities to resolve interpersonal deficiencies constellated in the transference, and it relies on the use of symbols and the theory of archetypes to facilitate children's understanding of their fears and fantasies. Through interpretation, Jungian play therapists link symbolic play with personal observations and relevant experiences in the child's external world as it relates to cultural and collective images and themes found in myths. One of the basic functions of myth is to help individuals through the journey of life, providing a travel guide to reach fulfillment—a map to discover "bliss." In interpretation, a therapist verbally acknowledges children's and adolescents' psychological maturation by applying larger themes of world mythology and identification with archetypal imagery to support transformation. In more concrete terms, Jungian play therapists rely upon verbal interventions (or well-timed reflections of meaning) that bridge connections between a child's unconscious (or inner landscape) and ancient symbols and modern art, mental illness or struggle and the hero's journey, thereby revealing the way myth helps identify one's heroic path (fig. 1.1).

The psyche's mythopoetic modes of reconstruction do not simply recreate ancient themes from fairy tales but rather destructively pull them apart and create new narratives on archetypal dynamics. This subversive process turns collective myths upside down and allows the child's psyche to remember what is long forgotten or censored or disfigured. Alchemists referred to this as "true imagination." Interpretation links embryonic forms of meaning as expressed in affect and symbolism to a specific life context, rendering it intelligible within a context beyond the personal unconscious. Once amplification occurs, the meaning of the symbol translates into the language of daytime consciousness and creates new affinities of meaning within the personal and the collective. Amplification as interpretation grounds children's images in mythologems, fairy tales, folklore, traditions, and customs. Interpretation amplifies the field of an image from the obscurely personal to the universal. It is numinous in that it reveals a child's personal connections between images and the archetypal or universal. The practical technique Fairy Tales in the Sand will help to concretize this complex information. This technique can be used by clinicians to connect children to their mythopoetic language.

Fairy Tales in the Sand, or FTS (Green, 2009a; Green & Gibbs, 2010) is a sand tray technique that connects children to the myths and mythopoetic language out of which the psyche leads to the healing. "Sand tray" differs from "sandplay" in that "sand tray" involves generic and theoretical application to sand work with children and the use of directive interventions, while sandplay is the Kalffian method that is based in Jung's theory and has no techniques necessarily. FTS recognizes archetypical displays in the child through fantasy imagery and fairy tale depictions. The FTS process begins by the therapist reading a fairy tale to the child. The therapist has four or five fairy tales to choose from, each possibly linked to some aspect of the child's current development or struggles. The child is then provided a simple, brief overview of the fairy tales and allowed to pick which one she wants to hear. After the child selects a fairy tale, the therapist reads the fairy tale and asks the child to identify a particularly important component of the fairy tale— an image, a theme, a plot, or a character. After the child has identified a

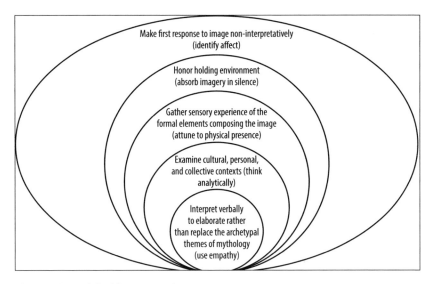

Figure 1.1. Model of interpretation

portion of the fairy tale, the child depicts the image or feeling associated with that symbol in the sand by creating a sand picture. The therapist silently observes while the child creates a picture in the sand. After the child finishes her original fairy tale sand picture, the therapist may discuss the scene with the child, by asking questions like, "Is there anything you'd like to share about your sand picture?" or "If you could give this sand picture a title, what would it be?" "Is there anything from this fairy tale that reminds you of anything at school or home, maybe?" FTS allows the child—through active imagination—to identify with myths and inherent archetypal realities that may provide numinous (spiritual) change. Specifically, children consciously connect to meaningful myths and mythical figures in fairy tales that carefully capture their personal struggles or the origin of their emotional predicament. Once children become aware of the myth and symbols that they are living out, they are able to more accurately form effective coping mechanisms to understand and transform pain and suffering into love and light.

Interventions

Though not an exhaustive list, the ideas below are cursory examples of Jungian play interventions with children. Most of these techniques are projective in nature, to cultivate a child's interior life, where a sense of depth and meaning are honored. These ideas are expounded in greater detail with clinical applications in later chapters.

Jungian Sandplay Therapy

Sandplay, developed by Dora Kalff (1980), typically involves a child playing in a sand tray and choosing sand miniatures to create a picture, with no direction or guidance and with little to no *processing* (resolving) afterward. Therapists permit children to draw, depict, or create whatever world they choose. The therapist may say, "Create a sand picture, and there's no right or wrong way to do this. After you finish, we may talk a little about your sand picture if you'd like. I'll be quiet while you play." After children finish creating their sand pictures, the therapist may say, "Is there anything you'd like to share about your sand picture? You don't have to if you don't want to—it's completely up to you."

If the mandala technique is to be used, the Jungian play therapist first asks the child to spend a couple of minutes relaxing. With eyes closed in a comfortable seated position, the child is led by the therapist through a guided imagery technique; the therapist helps the child to release any frustrations or anxieties accumulated throughout the school day through deep breathing. Also, the therapist may ask if the child wants to manipulate play dough or clay as an anxiety-releasing technique while breathing deeply. After a couple of minutes, the therapist asks the child to draw a large circle on a white piece of paper. The child is then instructed to depict, draw, or create a picture within the circle. Once the child finishes, the therapist and the child contemplate the images in silence. Jung (2008) believed the mandala, or an object (perhaps a circle) with an image contained within, represented unity or wholeness. From a Jungian perspective, unity or wholeness is commensurate with psychological healthiness, because, Jung believed, a reconciliation of opposites has occurred in the individual (*individuation*). In individuation, the child functions outside of the constraints of the ego, operating from the true center of being—the autonomous Self. Jungians believe that a mandala depiction is representative of the child's rich, interior life (Kalff, 1980).

Serial Drawings

Serial drawing is a technique in which a child produces images through various art media (mainly using colored pencils and plain white sheets of drawing paper) over a period of time, thus providing a projective or subjective assessment of the child's interior life to the therapist (Allan, 1988). After a therapeutic relationship and/or trust is formed between the therapist and the child, problems may be expressed symbolically (or sometimes concretely) in children's drawings. The serial drawing technique involves a therapist meeting with a child regularly and asking him to "draw a picture while we talk." Jung (1963) believed that in times of significant crisis, children could turn inward toward the unconscious for dreams and images that carried within them the potential for healing. Jung himself turned toward playing with stones by a lake for self-healing after his period of disorientation following the ideological break from Freud.

In serial drawings, the Jungian play therapist encourages the child to make the images independently by providing little to no instruction; permits the child to observe the images fully so that the Self can lead the child wherever he may need to go toward self-healing; and links the meaning of the symbols with the child's outer world at the point where the child's ego can accept and integrate the bridge between "transitional spaces." The serial drawing technique in itself does not heal, but rather provides the child a mechanism of safe expression and exploration of feelings associated with the psychological experience (Green & Hebert, 2006). While children move at their own pace, according to their developmental stages and available ego-energies to integrate conflicting or difficult emotions, typical designs in serial drawing technique have been observed by Allan (1988) and later slightly modified by Green (2008) into three central stages:

1. *Initial Stage* (first–fourth sessions): drawings
   — provide a glimpse of the child's interior, illustrated by symbols that reflect the source of trauma;
   — reflect the loss of internal or external control, with feelings of despair; and
   — establish initial rapport between the therapist and the child.
2. *Middle Stage* (fifth–eighth sessions): drawings reflect
   — a pure expression of intense emotion;
   — struggles between conflicting internal polarities (loss of control versus mastery); and
   — the deepening of the therapeutic relationship between the child and the therapist, which is exemplified by the child talking directly

about a traumatic issue or disclosing private and painful memories of the crisis to the therapist.

3. *Final Stage* (ninth–twelfth sessions): drawings reflect
   — images that reflect a sense of mastery, self-control, and valuation;
   — scenes with positive imagery;
   — a depiction of the Self (intact self-portraits or mandalas [circular shapes connoting wholeness/integration]);
   — scenes that are humorous with no macabre references; and
   — artwork representing autonomy from the therapeutic relationship.

In addition to open-mindedness for vagueness, therapists should offer an atmosphere that contains unconditional positive regard, trust, authenticity, warmth, and understanding, which may assist children to draw freely and produce unconscious symbol imagery through various media. To process (resolve) the serial drawing and amplify its symbols, Allan suggested that the therapist ask the child one or more of the following questions:

- Does this picture tell a story?
- I'm wondering if you can tell me what is happening in this scene?
- If you were inside this picture, what would it feel like?
- What went on in the story before this scene occurred? What happens next?
- Could you tell me what you were thinking or feeling as you drew this? (Allan, 1988)

During drawings, it is important for the therapist to remember that verbal and nonverbal communications to the child should reflect support, as in this way the child will come to realize that both good and horrible feelings are acceptable to convey in the therapeutic relationship.

Play Therapy Plan and Process

The JPT treatment plan has three steps: (1) counseling a child for 45 minutes twice per week in a controlled, emotionally and physically safe environment; (2) conducting one filial or family play therapy session with a child's family or caretakers every two to three weeks; and (3) regularly consulting with a multi-disciplinary team of school-based professionals to provide holistic care. Regarding the two sessions a week with a child in the consulting room, it may be helpful to the reader to have the JPT process fleshed out with a fuller context. The JPT process resembles that of the ancient alchemists. Alchemists (1400–1700) projected their internal processes into melding items of little value into something precious, such as iron into gold ("the philosopher's stone"). Also, alchemists believed that by converting base elements into spirit, the soul would be freed from its bodily prison. The alchemists always worked in relation to someone else to complete their mineral and spiritual transformations, referring to this "other" as the *soror mystica* (mystical sister). This is akin to conducting no play therapy without both an analyst and a child. The stages of the alchemical process inform the therapeutic aspects of the course of play therapy:

- *Fermentatio:* something is brewing up as the chemical reactions of the therapy process get under way. This involves changes in both the analyst and the child and is often seen at the onset of the psychotherapy;
- *Nigredo:* a blackening occurs because of the realization that imminent dangers lie ahead. We sometimes see this in children when they began to display highly reactive behaviors during therapy before they begin to stabilize;
- *Mortificato:* something must be extinguished and die. A change or shift in both the client and the therapist must occur before healing and containment begin.

Another conceptualization of the JPT process, one based on the heroic journey and archetypal theory, is presented in chapter 2.

The Role of the Therapist

The analytical play therapist's role is as an observer-participant (Allan, 1997). In practical terms, this means the clinician utilizes an integrative play therapy approach made up of nondirective play therapy (the child leads the play and does not receive direction from the therapist regarding what to do and when) along with more directive play therapy (the child uses therapist-introduced or therapist-invited techniques during play). It is part of the therapist's integrative philosophy to facilitate children's unearthing and incorporation of their shadow side to maintain psychic evenness or balance. The shadow is any aspect of the psyche that is excluded from conscious awareness. For example, a 12-year-old girl, Danita, was maltreated by her biological father as an infant. Danita exhibited a variety of symptoms, cognitions, and feelings in the playroom, including irrational fears of abandonment; attention-seeking, maladaptive behaviors; clinginess; and insecurity about the world around her. In Jungian terms, she was functioning out of a broken attachment complex, which could be treated by the therapist providing her psyche the freedom to enact these dysfunctional behaviors without judgment. Danita did indeed play out many scenes from her home life symbolically, using the playhouse, and the therapist provided interpretations throughout, with no criticism. She then internalized the good enough father imago within the transference with her therapist, as he provided examples of care and concern to her disturbing images. The father was seeking to make things right with his daughter and placed himself in individual counseling as well. They began rebuilding a relationship with each other. From this case, one may be able to infer that the psychotherapy process serves as a containment and a nurturing environment where the maternal or mother archetype activates through the transference to the therapist. After the child's psyche has an opportunity to display its broken and abandoned nature within an accepting and permissive atmosphere, the therapist introduces activities and interpretations and expresses genuine feelings of security, safety, and contentment. These interpretations provide a curative function so that the child's psyche may begin to fully realize and ultimately internalize the healing potential within herself.

The role of the Jungian play therapist includes making sense of symbols through an extensive process of personal analysis with a Jungian analyst; conceptualizing rage ego-syntonically (i.e., a broken attachment turns into rage and, if not remedied, depression and ultimately withdrawal) and helping children symbolize it; maintaining an analytical attitude that is both involved and detached; possessing the ability to direct children's raw material by carrying some of their psychological poison; and using sandplay, artwork, and dream analysis to amplify symbols and follow the child's Self wherever it leads (Green, 2009a, p. 91).

Finally, the central component of the play therapy relationship, in uniquely Jungian terms, is based upon this dialectic: interpersonal (observable behaviors and associated feelings) and intrapersonal (unconscious or inner drives) communication between analyst and child. Within the therapeutic exchanges, the analyst is just as much affected as the child. According to Samuels (2006), therapists must be flawed, recognize those flaws, and constructively work on those limitations in relation to the child. The therapist must accept that some of the child's interpretations are not merely transference projections but may be accurate assessments of the flaws within the therapist that need fixing. Jungian play therapists realize that the child needs opportunities to help or heal the therapist as well in this dynamic therapeutic relationship, so that the child's full developmental potential of healing others and herself may be realized.

The Role of the Caretaker

Parents or caretakers play a crucial role in the psychotherapy process with children. The play therapist needs to know what sort of transference is present and what is likely to develop in parents (Fordham, 1988). Therapists need the co-participation of parents throughout the counseling process. Depending upon the parents' psychopathology, a therapist may recommend that the mother or the father or both receive individual counseling from a different therapist. Parents are needed to manage any transitory regressions that may appear in the child during therapy, and their ego-strength must be bolstered to cope with this task. Therefore, many therapists incorporate parents into the play therapy process through either filial therapy or family play therapy. Typically, parent consultations and/or family play therapy is interwoven throughout the clinical process, perhaps every two to three weeks (but only after an initial period when the analyst and the child meet alone in the playroom to develop therapeutic rapport). It is not uncommon that the presenting problems initially observed in a child are not entirely remediated unless systemic attention is given to the relationship between the parents and the child and the family system as a monolithic functioning unit.

From a Jungian perspective, children play out the unconscious and unresolved conflicts within and between their parents. Jung (1963, 1964) believed that the unlived life of parents became the burden their children unconsciously carried. Furthermore, Jung stated that children introject the psychological and interpersonal discord of their parents. He believed that much of children's affect is determined by the quality of the relationship with their parents (Allan, 1997; Allan & Bertoia, 1992). For a more detailed perspective on incorporating caretakers in family play therapy with children, refer to Eliana Gil's book *Play in Family Therapy* (1994) or Charles Schaefer and Lois Carey's book *Family Play Therapy* (1994). Chapter 8 in this volume also provides additional details of including caretakers in the analytical play therapy process with children.

Conclusion

The central aim of JPT is for children to individuate. In common terminology this means children become more and more of who they really are, distinct from others (e.g., parents), yet learn about themselves in relation to others. The process is facilitated by a series of dialogues within the safety of a nonjudgmental therapeutic dyad where children uncover who they are in relation to the rest of the world through symbolic play (Green, 2009a). Once the unconscious is brought to the conscious level, mainly through sandplay, drawings, dream work, and amplifying symbols, children are less controlled by irrational forces and begin to mediate more rational behaviors aligned with the needs of a healthy ego. Through the transformation of affect (emotion) to image, the natural healing function of the child's psyche emerges. As Chodorow (2006) states, a child's imagination, constellated (activated) through spontaneous and symbolic play, replaces raw affect with images and stories that express the mood and emotion of the child more comprehensibly. The understanding of inner images and the associated feeling tones guides the process of psychological development. Finally, in the recently found *Red Book,* Jung (2009) states the importance and the healing nature of identifying the child archetype within himself during conflict toward the end of his life: "The spirit of the depths taught me that my life is encompassed by the divine child" (p. 234). Jung recognized the importance of the child archetype as compensating the one-sidedness of consciousness in adulthood and therefore facilitating psychological wholeness through a joining of opposites. Through interpretation, amplification, analysis, and connecting children to mythopoetic language through imagery in fairy tales and sandplay, the play therapist employs the micro-counseling skills involved in competently executing JPT.

2

Archetypes and Mythic Dimensions in
Child Psychotherapy

Now let me dare to open the wide gate
Past which men's steps have ever flinching trod . . .
Unpopular, ambiguous, and dangerous, it is a voyage of
discovery to the other pole of the world.

—Johann Wolfgang von Goethe

The purpose of this chapter is to provide a general overview of
theory from a post-Jungian perspective. It contains descriptive
data related to the works and theoretical concepts of Carl Jung applied to childhood development. Theory informs or underlies the
psychotherapeutic process. An overview of Jung's findings on archetypes is also included, to explain the salience of symbols as tools
for clinicians to utilize to lead children toward self-healing. Joseph
Campbell speaks about the myths individuals live out of, especially
during childhood. Recognizing these symbolic realities will educate
the mental health practitioner regarding the dynamic dimensions
correlated with psychological exploration in children. Briefly, theory provides the "why" in psychotherapy as techniques provide the
"what" as relationship provides the "how."

Jungian psychoanalysis has not been regarded traditionally in terms of its
application to children but primarily as a psychology of the adult. Specifically, Jung's theory centers on the second half of adult life, where he hypothesized that *individuation* (or becoming a *complete psychological individual*)
occurs. A complete psychological individual is one who is able to hold con-

flicting or polarizing emotions at once and not be inundated with distress by the contradictions; instead, the individual is able to exhibit healthy ego-functioning and engage in meaningful relationships with others. According to Main (2008), however, Jung viewed the child as a metaphorical image or archetype and focused on the psychology of "the child" or the symbol/myth inherent within the universal image of childhood. The archetype or image of "the child" is seen throughout Jung's early writings, especially in his *Theory of Psychoanalysis* (1913) and *Psychic Conflicts in a Child* (1910). In these writings, Jung reveals his views of childhood as being dependent upon caretakers. Through association tests, he demonstrated the far-reaching effects of identification between caretakers and children, so that a child's life is almost completely shaped by the unconscious or inner world of his parents.

Most of Jung's writings on children (2008) stemmed from his analysis of adult patients remembering their dreams from childhood, including the epic *somnia a deo missa* (dreams sent by God). He distilled that much of the underlying psychological content in these dreams from childhood was related to parents' psychopathology. It was not until much later in his studies that he began the process of applying his notion of archetypes to childhood. Eventually, his theory became vulnerable to derision. Specifically, critics were discontent with the soundness of Jung's esoteric theory unless archetypes could be observed in childhood and throughout the lifespan, not exclusively in the latter part of adulthood.

For Jung, "the child" does not refer to the human child but essentially refers to the universal symbol or archetype of the child, found in myths, fairy tales, dreams, and fantasies (Fordham, 1994a; Jung, 1951; Main, 2008). Jung was not interested in the child's development, necessarily, but more in the myth-making function of the psyche during childhood. He found that the archetype of the child appears in various child motifs, since an archetype by definition cannot be directly described, such as "the eternal child, "the divine child," and "the child of chaos." Two commonalities in Jung's symbolic view of childhood across all motifs involve *autonomy* and *spontaneity*.

Jung was one of Freud's disciples at the turn of the twentieth century, defending Freud's radical psychoanalytic theory with its heavy emphasis on the psychosexual and irrational nature of the psyche. In 1913, Jung resigned as president of Freud's International Psychoanalytic Association because he had come to disagree with Freud's sexual trauma theory. He saw delusions as archetypes, not repressed memories as Freud postulated, and published his disagreements in *Symbols of Transformation* in 1916. Following the public and humiliating break from Freud, Jung experienced a protracted period of isolation during which he wrote volumes about the collective unconscious and the process of individuation. Jung's last book before his death, *Man and His Symbols,* illustrated his focus in the last part of his life on the intersectionalities between culture, spirituality, and archetypes. His ideas served as the foundation for the Myers-Briggs Type Indicator, a commonly utilized personality inventory, and have influenced play therapy with children, art therapy, and the integration of the symbolic life in psychotherapy.

Wanting to explore the analytical process with children, Jung encouraged Dora Kalff (1980) to study under Margaret Lowenfield and develop a method for symbolic play in child therapy, which she later termed *sandplay*. Starting in the 1930s, Melanie Klein (1955), a child psychoanalyst, influenced by Jung's work, developed a revolutionary approach to working with children, including the use of play techniques. Inspired by Klein, Jungian analyst Michael Fordham (1994b) wrote *The Life of Childhood*, where it was argued, for the first time with evidence from actual child analysis and not simply from analyses of adults, as Jung had previously attempted to do, that archetypes were observable in children and were a significant component in the therapeutic process. Archetypes refer to the predisposition to create images, to organize experience, and to determine an individual's relationship between the inner and outer worlds. Fordham goes on to say that the archetypal content in children is related to drives, instincts, and bodily experiences in relation to the child's mental world. Development and psychological maturation lead the child toward the spiritual end of the archetype, where he can cultivate individuality and engage in collective thinking.

Later, Sidoli and Davies (1988) refined Jung's theory and adapted it to children in a book titled *Jungian Child Psychotherapy*. John Allan went on to refine the theory of Jungian child psychotherapy further by the specificity of incorporating play therapy techniques in child analysis, with various applications, through his seminal book *Inscapes of the Child's World* (1988). Recently, authors J. P. Lilly (2009), Gisela De Domenico (1994), J. Craig Peery (2003), and Eric Green (2007, 2008, 2009a, 2009b) have continued to write, provide trainings at national conferences, and practice Jungian Play Therapy with children and families. The next section provides an overview of the analytical and archetypal theory of development in children's personalities.

The Development of the Child's Personality

Carl Gustav Jung was born on July 26, 1875, in Kesswyl, Switzerland. His father was a Protestant minister, in whom Jung identified personality flaws, based on his perceptions that his father was unable to effectively convey and practice the faith he preached. Jung's disenchantment with his father's spirituality was the genesis of Jung's lifelong search for his own religion, eventually culminating in the erudite theory eponymously titled Jungian analytical psychology. The relationship to the symbolic life, or how individuals relate to the symbols inside themselves, was the crux of Jung's theory of *individuation,* a lifelong inner journey of self-discovery and transformation. Jung postulated that growth happens when one works with symbols in dreams and follows the symbols wherever they lead. Jung's psychology centers on the contrast of descent, going down into the underworld, and the natural ascent back to the external world.

With its origins in psychoanalytic theory, Jungian Play Therapy focuses on the psyche's role in child personality development (Klein, 1955). *Psyche* is defined as the child's center of thought that regulates conscious experiences, such as behaviors and feelings. Jung (1963) explained the evolving nature of the child's psyche in accordance with the collective unconscious and how it influences the process of individuation. Jung's concept of the collective unconscious was less person-specific than Freud's concept of the *unconscious,* and it was "identical in all men and thus constitutes a common psychic substrate of a suprapersonal nature which is present in every one of us" (Jung, 1959, p. 4). Individuation is characterized as a progress from psychic fragmentation toward wholeness—the acknowledgment and reconciliation of opposites within an individual (Jung, 1963).

Jung (1959, 1964) supplanted Freud's theory of a personal unconscious— a depository of individual unconscious memories and repressed emotions— with a *collective unconscious* consisting of universal images that transcend an individual's personal (or conscious) experience. The collective unconscious consists of primordial images and mythological motifs often manifested in fairy tales, Greek myths, and ancient legends. Jung compared Freud's concept of the personal unconscious as an individual-specific, encapsulated fragment of a human's personality and intimate life to his concept of the collective unconscious. Jung disagreed with psychoanalytic theory, discounting the potency of basic biological and irrational needs. Jungian theory describes the instinctive yearnings in humans as soulful and archetypal remnants that are motivated by a psycho-spiritual proclivity for growth and evolution. Moreover, Jung believed humans have a capacity for conscious self-growth through innate symbols, or archetypes. Fordham (1994a) took this a step further and stated that childhood, not just the latter part of adult life as Jung stated, is a time of individuation. In children, the growth process revolves around the ego separating from the Self, and in later adulthood, growth occurs from the re-integration and alignment of the Self with the ego. While the conscious mind makes up the ego, the child's unconscious mind consists of the collective unconscious and the personal unconscious. The personal unconscious is a repository of repressed memories, fantasies, wishes, traumas, and desires that accumulate over the course of an individual's lifespan. Within the personal unconscious exists the shadow, which carries both the benevolent and the malevolent portions of the personality. Jung believed that by integrating the shadowy aspects of the personality through analysis, psychic healing and wholeness could occur.

Jung believed that at birth there was no ego consciousness; he saw ego as the center of the conscious mind. Jung stated that the ego is embedded in the Self. At birth, ego de-integrates, exemplified by eye moving, the calming of a distressed infant, sucking, being comforted, and crying, all of which form ego. De-integration of the ego is followed by re-integration if the infant is comforted by a caretaker. When the child is adequately cared for (i.e., fed when hungry, held when scared, diaper changed regularly), positive parental introjects, or imagoes, emerge, creating a sense of secure attachment. With secure attachment, children are positioned to develop healthy coping skills and ego-strength to resolve adverse emotional events. In some instances, the infant's primal needs are not mediated by a caretaker, and the infant introjects negative images of the mother and father imagoes. These negative images are internalized as not good enough parents, which create rigid ego defenses (Allan, 1997). Ego defenses become rigid because they must protect the child's fragile ego from annihilation owing to the myriad feelings of abandonment, rejection, and desolation. Additionally, Jung stated that the infant was no empty slate: the psyche carries contrasexual images. Men carry the anima (female traits) and women carry the animus (male traits). Together the anima and the animus form a *hieros gamos,* a union representing the union of polarities within the personality, exemplified by the yin and yang in Eastern religions, or Adam and Eve from the Christian biblical story of creation.

There are four functions of a child's psychology that resolve how the child perceives internal and external stimuli that shade the child's personality: (1) *Sensation* is perceiving through physical stimuli and is categorized by people who are concrete; (2) *Thinking* involves cognitive processing and utilizing intellect to analyze and interpret; (3) *Intuition* bases perceptions on "gut" feelings in contrast to sensate functioning; and (4) *Feeling*, the opposite of thinking, is where emotions and values are prominent (Seligman, 2006). In addition to those four functions, Jung postulated that two attitudes exist for children to perceive the world. *Introverts* reflect from within their inner world and accumulate strength in solitude. *Extroverts* first examine the external stimuli, then relate these stimuli to their interior life, gaining energy from socializing with other people.

Trauma: Developmental Disruptions

An infant's ego defenses rely upon nascent defensive structures that create breaks in the hypothetical *ego-Self axis* when an infant's physiological and emotional needs are inadequately supported. The *ego-Self axis* is a Jungian term for the negotiation between the child's inner and outer worlds (Allan, 1997). With the introjection of the *bad parent image,* the child may recognize the world as dangerous and unbalanced. With this insecure attachment come feelings of degradation and being *not good enough* (Winnicott, 1971). Because of the nascent functioning of the ego in early childhood, rigid ego defenses develop to protect the insubstantial ego, which creates a psychopathology of defensive splitting of the Self from the ego for preservation (Green, 2009a).

A child's autonomous personality may encounter disrepair when faced with an imminent, sustained level of hyper-arousal or extreme traumatic anxiety (Jung, 1964). Kalsched (1996) speculated that, to avoid this eradication, an *archetypal self-care system* comes to the child's aid—an archaic mechanism that creates a defensive splitting to encapsulate the child's delicate personal spirit in safety by banishing it to the unconscious. The child's psychic defense against insufferable pain sends an archetypal *daimon,* or an image from the self-care system, to protect the child's *transitional space.* According to Kalsched (1996), the transitional space is the realm between the inner and the outer world where the child learns how to play creatively and utilizes symbols. Traumatic anxiety interrupts the transitional space and may temporarily quench the child's capacity to be imaginative through symbolic play.

For the child's ego to resolve the effects of trauma, a meaningful *integration* must occur. Meaning, according to Kalsched (1996), occurs when children's bodily excitations are given mental representation by transitional archetypal figures so that they eventually can reach verbal or symbolic expression and be shared with a trusting, caring individual. Helping the child recover the tenuous transitional space, so that her creative capacities are restored, entails the enhancement of the connection between the unconscious and the conscious (Allan, 1988; Jung, 1963). This results in strengthening the child's ego and its capacity to explore polarities that are both painful and comforting (e.g., anger/forgiveness, pride/humility, aggressiveness/assertiveness). From a Jungian perspective, this *coniunctio oppositorum,* or a joining of opposites, portrayed in the child's drawing, painting, or verbalization of symbolic images from dreams or the unconscious in the presence of a nonjudgmental, empathic therapist facilitates psychological healing.

Theoretical Underpinnings of Jungian Play Therapy Treatment Stages

The Jungian Play Therapy process resembles the mythic journey of the *hero* as articulated by Joseph Campbell (2008). The hero's journey involves individuals who are placed involuntarily into a situation or journey that is typically against their will and not of their choosing (e.g., parents typically bring their child to a therapist; seldom does a child ask to receive counseling). The circumstances surrounding the individual embarking on this journey are typically adverse and aberrant (e.g., children are typically brought to therapy because they are struggling with depression, rage, emptiness, defiance, psychosis). The hero travels a long, epic journey, often through a dark, perilous forest (e.g., the child sets out on an extended therapeutic experience, typically lasting a year or so, with difficult feelings emerging along the way). The dangerous middle ground is filled with confusion, detours, primal fears, and evil beings.

The hero combats the nefarious elements along the way and perseveres through the forest, seeking a magic elixir or some type of potion to resolve the unfortunate issue(s) that catapulted him to the beginning of the journey (e.g., the child is led by the Self to produce symbols and resolve ego conflicts). The hero can identify that she is on this great odyssey if she is visited by fairies, a wise old sage, or some type of guide that delivers advice along the way to help her reach her destination (e.g., the play therapist). For example, the character Gollum in J. R. R. Tolkien's novel *The Lord of the Rings* was Frodo's guide through the enchanted forest to his final destination, Mordor. The hero's journey is not complete until the hero retrieves the potion or new knowledge and returns to his village or home and tells others about it, sharing the knowledge or integrating what he learned from the trip (e.g., successful termination happens after the child's ego-Self axis has strengthened and her self-acceptance and social relationships improve).

Specifically, the Jungian treatment process is cyclical and not linear. However, it can be codified generally into three stages: orientation, working-through, and reparation/termination. During the orientation phase, the therapist builds an alliance with the child by establishing the frame (i.e., a consistent time and weekday in specific space), purpose (i.e., playing, talking about worries, sharing dreams), and conditions or limits of therapy (Allan, 1997; Allan & Brown, 1993; Green, 2009a). Here is an example of the *orientation* phase between "Andrew" and his play therapist as they begin the play therapy process:

> *Andrew*: What should I do first?
>
> *Dr. Green*: Andrew, that's something you can decide. In here, you can play with all of the toys in most of the ways you want. Every Tuesday and Friday from 4:00 pm–4:45 pm, in this room, will be our special playtime. And whichever parent brings you to our playtime will remain in the waiting room outside the playroom door until we are done. The reason why I play with children in here is because sometimes kids may have worries and don't know how to express them. Sometimes playing helps.
>
> *Andrew*: My brother says I get angry sometimes, but I don't get scared. I don't get scared like my sister does sometimes in the dark.
>
> *Dr. Green*: You see yourself as brave (providing an interpretation).
>
> *Andrew* (smiles): Yes, I'm very brave. Now watch how I make this airplane fly.

In the *working-through* phase, the child's negative behavioral and personality traits appear and transference occurs, during which emotional woundedness, introjections of negative parental imagoes, and rage materialize (De Domenico, 1994). It is of paramount importance that therapists accept the shadow side of children and acknowledge its presence in the playroom. "The monstrous, destructive, and catabolic elements of the personality need free expression while being securely held by the therapist in a benign, nontraumatizing way" (p. 272). Often the thematic content of children's play in the working-through phase resembles the natural cycles of life, with death and rebirth, damnation and salvation, and hatred and love ubiquitously interwoven. The following excerpt is from Andrew's sixth session.

Andrew: And the evil dragon would kill everyone and everything in burning fire!!

Dr. Green: The dragon wants everyone to know how powerful he is!

Andrew (screams): Yes, and stop talking, or he'll burn you too! (he starts throwing sand out of the sandtray and all over the room, chaotically).

Dr. Green (breaks the metaphor and interprets to de-escalate): Andrew, I'm wondering if you ever feel like the dragon in that sand picture and you get tired of people telling you what you can and can't do?

Andrew: YES!! And I will kill everyone if they don't realize how powerful I am! (pauses). Sorry, Mr. Green. I didn't really mean I would kill you or anyone. I'm just playing.

Dr. Green: Sometimes I say things when I'm upset too that I maybe don't mean. And in here, it's OK to express your feelings. It's OK to get mad in here.

Andrew: OK. Where's the vacuum? Wanna help me clean up?

Dr. Green: Sure, tell me what you'd like for me to do.

From a Jungian perspective, violence is a defense against pain, as aggression is a defense against sadness. The therapist recognized that the child's ego was leading him straight to *the wounding*. Because the therapist recognized this movement, he did not stop the feeling. Allan (1988) and Allan and Clark (1984) stated that the more psychological poison the child releases (descent), the better the recovery (ascent). Through the therapist's interepretations and acceptance of all parts of Andrew's personality exhibited behaviorally and symbolically in the playroom, Andrew moved deeper into the analytical process. From a Jungian perspective, if a child wants to change the rage, he must enter the rage. This is a hallmark of the *working-through* phase.

During the *reparation and termination* phase, children often depict circles, or mandalas, in their drawings and sandplay. Following is a brief excerpt of this final phase between Andrew and this play therapist toward the end of their time together:

Andrew: This is the circle of light (pointing to a circular shape he made in the sand tray with jewels). And in this circle everyone is loved.

Dr. Green: What could you do, in your own life, to create your own circle of power? (interpreting and connecting inner to outer realities).

Andrew: Maybe I could let my family love me, and love them back.

Through connecting the circle of life or mandala from his sand picture, Andrew developed the capacity to find caring feelings and behaviors toward himself and others. Through play, he managed the tensions between the opposites and feels better about the world and his place in it. The emotionally and physically safe, trusting, nonjudgmental therapeutic relationship, along with the *temenos* or sacred space within the playroom and the analytical attitude of the therapist, orchestrated to activate the archetype of *containment*. According to Jungian Play Therapy, containment of emotions is integral as a part of the final stage in play therapy and beyond.

Conclusion

Jungian Play Therapy and its theoretical underpinnings from analytical psychology as outlined in this chapter render several important implications. First, play therapists should consistently be in therapy themselves with a trained analyst or depth-psychologist. Because there is such a commingling of personalities between analyst and child, especially with the analyst therapeutically *carrying* or *holding* the child's maladjustment, there is a real and probable risk that the child's projections may contaminate the analyst's psyche. Play therapists *take over* the suffering of children; and in doing so, they may have their own psychological sicknesses activated outside the playroom or unconsciously transferred onto the child inside the playroom. Jung (1951) stated, "If he [the therapist] feels that the patient is hitting him, even scoring off of him: it is his own hurt that gives the measure of this power to heal" (p. 116). From a Jungian standpoint, therapists may make right in their patients only what they have made right within themselves. In essence, the play therapist must change as much as the child does for therapy to be effective.

The second theoretical implication from Jung's theory as applied to play therapy is that children are viewed as sensitive human beings that need someone to simply *be* with them for a short time, and not viewed as dysfunctional objects in need of a standardized, cold, clinical cure. This implies the salience and the centerpiece of psychotherapy: the nonjudgmental therapeutic alliance. For Jungians it is the most crucial variable when facilitating change in children's self-healing. Children will not remember all of the elegant interpretations, sophisticated techniques, or accurate empathic responses, necessarily, when they think back on the special time with their play therapist. Children remember the kindness we show them (Green, 2009a).

A third implication from theory, as articulated in the stages of play therapy, is that children need to know, from the very beginning, that they set the pace, direction, and tone of counseling. And more importantly, they can place their trust in a caring adult who will be with them, not against them. Of fundamental importance is that play therapists make a therapeutic connection to children in need, by accepting them for who they are without trying to change what they are. Throughout psychotherapy, the play therapist *absorbs* and *contains* children's inner longings and desires, pain and sadness, murderous fantasies and destructive impulses, jealousy and tumultuous rage, and inner strength and resiliency.

II JUNGIAN PLAY THERAPY

Interventions

3

Sandplay

To the extent that I managed to translate the emotions into images, I was inwardly calmed and reassured. Had I left those images hidden in the emotions, I might have been torn to pieces by them.

—Carl Jung

———

Jungian analyst Dora Kalff's term *sandplay* was rooted in the premise of Jung's belief that the psyche can be activated to move toward wholeness and healing, and that individuation occurred in the sand process through the *temenos,* or free and protected space. The clinician provides the free and protected space in which a creation in the sand may symbolize the inner drama and healing potential of the child's psyche. The protected space refers to the way the therapist listens, observes, and serves nonjudgmentally as a psychological container for the emotional content that becomes activated by the sand therapy process. Activating the self-healing force in a child's psyche to resolve psychosocial struggles will occur only within the safety of the space where unconscious forces are free to reproduce, as is inherent in sandplay. This chapter includes a case study of sandplay with a child diagnosed with an externalizing behavioral disorder.

Jungian sandplay originated in the 1950s when Jung asked Swiss psychotherapist Dora Kalff to study sandplay under Margaret Lowenfeld in London. In the 1920s, Lowenfeld (1979) had developed a therapeutic method for preschool children to communicate their feelings and thoughts, symbolically, by playing in sand. Through the use of sand trays, sand, and sand miniatures, Lowenfeld discovered that children communicated conscious and unconscious thoughts in less threatening ways than by directly verbalizing them to an adult. Lowenfeld created the *world technique,* a therapeutic intervention in which children used sand figurines in a sand tray to construct a world.

In 1962, Kalff built on Lowenfeld's work and termed the intervention *sandplay* while at a conference of Jungian analysts in California (Steinhardt, 2000). Kalff's (1980) sandplay was rooted in Jung's belief that the psyche can be activated to move toward wholeness and healing and that individuation occurs in the sand process through the *temenos,* or free and protected space. *Protected space* refers to the way in which the therapist listens, observes, and serves nonjudgmentally as a psychological container for the emotional content that becomes activated by the sand therapy process (Green, 2008; McNulty, 2007). The therapist provides the free and protected space in which a creation in the sand may symbolize the inner drama and healing potential of the child's psyche. The therapeutic space is referred to in the literature by multiple names, including *secured symbolizing field* (Goodheart, 1980), *transitional play space* (Winnicott, 1971), and *third area* or *area of experience* (Gordon, 1993). Activating the self-healing force in a child's psyche to resolve psychosocial struggles may occur within the safety of the space where unconscious forces are free to reproduce, as is inherent in sandplay.

Rationale

The therapeutic rationale for sandplay is that children reproduce symbolic scenes of their immediate experience and link opposites from their inner and outer worlds. Through the concretization of unconscious experiences, children's psyches are able to make meaningful links and develop mastery over difficult feelings. Moreover, it is what children experience for themselves that is therapeutic in sandplay (Bradway & McCoard, 2005; De Domenico, 1994), not the therapist's analysis of the symbols contained within the scene. The emerging worlds in the tray illustrate the child's unconscious conflicts as sandplay provides an opportunity for both symbolic and realistic grounding to occur. Moreover, sandplay permits children to express their archetypal and intrapersonal worlds, connects them to everyday reality, and creates a communication between the conscious and unconscious minds through which psychogenic healing occurs (Boik & Goodwin, 2000; Carey, 1999; Green & Connolly, 2009).

Themes

Themes or symbols emerge out of children's sandplay. These themes are typically fluid, serving as guides for further exploration when a child is assisted within the therapeutic context. Steinhardt (2000) listed meanings of symbols in sandplay. The meanings were meant to be guideposts or generalities for the therapist, not static definitions, because symbols and their meanings differ among individuals. All symbols in sandplay should be carefully viewed in the context of the individual child and the meaning the child ascribes to them. Steinhardt described the following symbols that may appear in sandplay:

- a hole scooped out of the sand could symbolize a cave, a womb, a volcano, or an entrance into the collective unconscious;
- a mound in the sand or a mountain could symbolize the body of the Earth Mother, a container of warmth;
- lines drawn in the sand could be seen as a life path, a demarcation of territory, or a new path to follow;
- a tunnel or a bridge could symbolize communication between where one is and where one wants to go or has been;
- passages downward could symbolize burying something hideous to the conscious or the shadow; and
- resurrection of buried objects may symbolize repressed emotions being released or exposed.

One of the most common sand activities in which children engage is burying objects (Steinhardt, 2000). Children enjoy burying small objects in the sand tray, just as they enjoy burying objects in sand while playing on a beach. Sometimes children will ask their therapist to find the object hidden in the sand tray. Jungian-oriented counselors could view this request in several different ways. First, children's search into the sand's depth could symbolize the belief that their inner world could be unearthed with the therapist's help. Second, children's request for the therapist to locate hidden objects in the sand tray may be viewed as the children's revealing something that had been unclear or scary and that can now be revealed and tolerated without judgment. Third, the burial of an object could symbolize children's longing for self-acceptance or parental approval, buried deep within their unconscious longings and tacit desires. Or the child could be simply be having fun burying objects in the sand, with no deeper subtext involved.

Process

When introducing sandplay, play therapists may say, "Here are two trays filled with sand. As you can see, one tray is wet; the other tray is dry. . . . Would you like to feel the sand?" Then, "Here (gesturing to shelves of miniatures) are small, miniature toys and other objects you can use in the sand trays (table 3.1). If you like, you can use these objects to make a picture in the sand." Later, if the client does create a sand picture, sandplay therapists often add, "After you leave today, I am going to take a picture of what you've made in the sand, if that is all right with you, so you can later see all of your sandplay pictures." Usually children do not ask to see pictures of their "old" sandplay trays; they are busy creating new aspects of their lives. However, child clients may return as adults to review their sandplay pictures (Mitchell et al., 2014).

Sandplay therapy, within the context of play therapy, allows a child to create an imaginative world by placing miniatures in a tray (19.5 x 28.5 with a depth of 3 inches), half-filled with fine-grained, sterilized white sand and painted blue on the inside to give the impression of water and/or sky. Dora Kalff (1980), the founder of sandplay therapy, said that sand represents instinct, nature, and the healing power of Mother Earth. The miniatures on nearby shelves are a stimulus to the child's imagination and represent many aspects in the child's world. The child's choice of miniatures helps the therapist to symbolically understand the issues that are displayed in the sand (Mitchell et al., 2014).

Normally, two trays are available in sandplay therapy, so the child will have a choice of wet (damp) sand or dry sand. A container of water is often nearby so that more water can be added to the sand. Sandplay serves as a window into the client's inner world; it provides the opportunity to express a myriad of feelings, unspoken thoughts, and even the unknown. Sandplay pictures may be created quickly, in ten minutes or so, or may take the entire therapeutic hour. Usually, a sandplay picture is not created at every therapy session; it is the child's choice when, and whether, to use sandplay (Mitchell et al., 2014).

After giving the child an opportunity to examine the toys and miniatures during the first session, some therapists ask, "Would you like to make a picture in the sand now?" The reason for inviting the child to create a sand

Table 3.1. Examples of Jungian sand tray miniatures

Category	Examples
People	Adults and children of different ethnicities, religious figures, heroes and villains, brides and grooms, occupational and sports figures
Animals	Zoo and domestic birds, insects, sea life
Infrastructure	Houses, churches, schools, castles, bridges, buildings
Vehicles	Cars, trucks, airplanes, boats, motorcycles, ambulances, police cars
Vegetation	Trees, bushes, flowers
Boundaries	Fences, gates, barricades
Fantasy	Witches, wizards, wishing wells, treasure chests, unicorns, dragons, fairies, crystal balls, magical jeweled stones
Spiritual	Angels, demons, priests, shamans, totem poles, star of David, Torah, Bible, doves
Nature	Rainbows, sun, moon, stars, mountains, rocks, caves, trees, bushes, flowers, water
Practical items	Household furniture, such as toilets, bathtubs; desks, pens, shovels
Miscellaneous	Wine and beer bottles, jewelry, guns, knives, wrapped gifts

picture during the first or second therapy session is that playing in the sand will often help the child feel more comfortable in the new play therapy environment. In addition, the content of the tray and the process the child uses in creating a sand picture can provide useful information about the child. For example, Kalff (1980) said that a first tray may suggest (a) how the child feels about therapy, (b) the child's relationship to the unconscious, (c) the nature of the problem, or (d) the solution to the problem. In our experience, the first tray can also give information about the child's relationship to the therapist. Also, because children under 8 years old tend to create trays similar to those created by other children of the same age, it is possible to acquire a deeper understanding of the child's developmental level from the child's first sandplay creation, especially if the tray deviates from the norm (Mitchell et al., 2014).

Benefit

From a Jungian perspective, sandplay is the physical embodiment of active imagination. It frees creativity, perceptions, inner feelings, and memories as the child transports unconscious thoughts and feelings from the interior to the exterior realm of consciousness directly to the sand tray. Second, many children view sandplay as a natural form of expression, and they are readily attracted to it. Although some children are reticent to engage in certain play activities (i.e., some children are resistant to undertake art activities because they do not believe that they are good artists), they tend to respond positively to sandplay because they feel free to create with less self-criticism or constraint (Green & Christensen, 2006). Third, sandplay is a technique that facilitates a sense of mastery over difficult feelings and conflicted thoughts. Moreover, because sandplay involves nonverbal expression, it engenders a necessary therapeutic distance from distressing or traumatic events for children, including the engagement in disordered or disruptive behaviors.

Sandplay is distinguished from other forms of therapy: it permits children to create a picture that provides concrete images of their inner thoughts and feelings, because the symbols and sand miniatures serve as a common language. Also, sandplay provides a unique kinesthetic quality because the extremely tactile experience of manipulating sand can be a therapeutic encounter. Touching and playing in the sand may produce a calming effect in anxious or disruptive preschool children (Shih et al., 2006). From a Jungian perspective, the primary therapeutic benefit of sandplay involves the autonomous and regenerative healing power of the child's psyche, which activates and produces symbols that are witnessed without judgment by a caring therapist. Kalff (1980) emphasized that the transformative experience of creating a picture in the sand contains the healing. Sandplay facilitates healing and transformation in young children by releasing conflicts from the unconscious in symbolic form and by supporting a healthy reordering of psychological contents (Turner, 2005).

Finally, sandplay therapists believe that children's creative expressions in the sand exemplify a cathartic release of their current distress, pathology, grief, hope, or all of these. Moreover, sandplay shows the mechanism by which children are coping with emotional pain and wounding. By expressing their psychogenic pain in the sand tray, children participate in an emotional catharsis, which may release repressed hostilities and rage associated with unconscious conflicts at the root of disruptive behaviors. "Each sand tray in the process may be seen as part of a series of successive attempts to cope with past and current wounds or as a step in the ongoing journey towards individuation or, almost necessarily, both" (Bradway & McCoard, 2005, p. 49). Catharsis is facilitated by the witnessing of the child's sand scenes by a nonevaluative, caring, trusted adult.

Case Illustration

Tyler, a 5-year-old boy, was referred to counseling by the headmistress at the preschool he was attending. On the day of the referral, Charlotte, Tyler's mother, was asked to pick up her son from his preschool. According to the headmistress, Tyler was being disobedient and wanted to play aggressively with other children instead of completing his school tasks. Because of his disruptive behavior, he was not permitted to return to the school until he met with a child psychotherapist and a pediatrician.

Because of the child's age, Tyler's mother was referred to a play therapist (the author of this book). After the initial intake with Charlotte, the play therapist consulted with a variety of significant adults in Tyler's life to formulate a clinical picture and procure an accurate diagnosis. Labels and diagnoses are important only in that they incorporate evidence-based practices and maintain accountability to patients when third-party payers are involved. After procuring the necessary releases of confidential information, the play therapist consulted with the headmistress, who provided the following biographical information about Tyler. She stated that Tyler had been born and raised in a highly dysfunctional family and that his father was often verbally and physically abusive toward Charlotte. She said that Tyler had lived in several shelters and presented a socially deviant temperament because of inconsistencies in his home life. She also mentioned that Charlotte occasionally spanked Tyler and that teachers at Tyler's previous preschool spanked him as well because of his disobedient behaviors. She said he was defiant, hit and punched children, threatened children with violence, used inappropriate language, spat on children, shoved other children, and lacked empathy.

As part of the cognitive behavioral intake, the therapist uncovered the following information about Tyler from his mother, his mother's boyfriend, his grandparents, and his teachers. Tyler had witnessed domestic violence at a very young age, perhaps as early as 6 months old, according to his mother. Tyler's father engaged in regular drinking binges, had low self-esteem, lacked empathy for others, was highly aggressive, stole jewelry and valuables out of people's homes to make extra income, lacked friendships, and regularly vandalized and damaged other people's property. He regularly physically abused his wife while Tyler watched. When he was 4 years old, Tyler made the following comment to Charlotte after witnessing his father beating her with a leather belt: "I want to die 'cause no one loves me."

Charlotte moved out of her home with her son to escape the domestic violence and precarious situation she believed her son was in with her abusive and alcoholic husband. Consequently, she and Tyler had moved among 12 different shelters, halfway houses, cities, and schools before Tyler was 5 years old. Many of the caretakers in Tyler's life had commented on his anger, rage, and disruptive behaviors, citing incidences of his failure to follow household or school rules, repetitively arguing or reasoning, propensity to challenge authority figures, talking excessively at inappropriate times, frequent interruptions, difficulty waiting his turn, and impulsivity. His mother and grandparents noted that he displayed the following traits with chronicity: stubbornness, hyper-distractibility, overactivity, and aggressiveness. In the six months before his referral, Tyler had developed the following new temperaments: suspicious cautiousness, frequent temper outbursts, impulsiveness, and violence. A multi-disciplinary team consisting of a pediatrician, a neurologist, a psychiatrist, and a play therapist diagnosed Tyler with Oppositional Defiant Disorder and Attention-Deficit/Hyperactivity Disorder, combined type.

Analytical Conceptualization

From a Jungian perspective, when an unbearable level of anxiety devastates the child's susceptible ego, as in the case of Tyler's witnessing his mother being verbally abused and physically beaten or as when his mother was physically aggressive with him, *de-integration* occurs and threatens to annihilate the child's personality (Green, 2008, 2009a; Jung, 1964). Kalsched (1996) theorized that to prevent this eradication, an archetypal self-care system comes to the child's rescue. This is an antiquated apparatus that creates a defensive splitting to encapsulate the child's fragile personal spirit in safety by expelling it to the unconscious. The child's psychic defense against unendurable pain sends an archetypal *daimon,* or an image from the self-care system, to help the child detach from the vast anxiety (Green, 2008, 2009a). Children who, like Tyler, exhibit severe externalizing behavior problems often have a *disconnect* between the Self and their ego's stability in managing the external world. Specifically, children with aggressive and disruptive behavior problems may have particularly deprived links between their inner and outer worlds because of the deterioration of their good-enough parental *introjects* (i.e., the images and feelings associated with those images of the good mother or good father archetypes that provide safety). Tyler's *good-enough parent image* dissolved when he watched his father persistently and savagely abuse his mother and when she physically disciplined him.

As implied by the quote Charlotte provided from Tyler regarding wanting to die and feeling unloved, young children who witness chronic domestic violence or who are on the receiving end of corporal punishment may feel rejected at a profoundly deep, primal level because they personalize the attacks and wonder, "What's wrong with me? Why am I not OK?" Tyler developed aggressive and disruptive behaviors to (a) mediate the immense anxiety he experienced from witnessing domestic violence and receiving harsh physical discipline; (b) seek attention from significant caretakers, whether positive or negative, to recover from his feelings of being not good enough; (c) cope, in a primal or rudimentary way, with his feelings of intense sadness, dejection, and uprootedness resulting from his and his mother's frequent moves; and (d) model his parents' behaviors of coping with extreme stress.

Treatment Goals

Helping Tyler recover his good-enough parent imago so that his creative capacities would be reestablished would involve the augmentation of the link between the unconscious and the conscious (Allan, 1988; Green, 2008; Jung, 1963). In Jungian sandplay, this entails increasing Tyler's ego strength and its capacity to explore emotional polarities (e.g., hatred-forgiveness, desolation-connectedness, and terror-safety) arising within the safety of the sand tray projections. Jungian Play Therapy penetrates deep psychic mechanisms by exploring emotional polarities or complexes, and sandplay allows for the release of rage associated with the painful and shadowy aspects of these emotional polarities. Once the child's psyche has the opportunity to become cognizant of and release the indefatigable feelings of suffering through sandplay, breaks in the defensive wall of the ego may emerge that stimulate self-healing.

The sandplay treatment goals with Tyler included (a) building an emotionally safe, trusting, therapeutic alliance in which he could self-nurture and internalize a positive, good-enough parental imago; (b) allowing for the expression of complicated emotions through representational and tangible channels and regulating or achieving mastery over these difficult emotions; (c) giving his rage a voice in the playroom and therapeutically carrying that rage so that it could be altered; (d) conducting family play therapy sessions with Charlotte every two to three weeks to provide different ways of interacting with her son that would decrease disruptive behaviors; and (d) collaborating with Tyler's preschool teacher and school counselor to provide regular mental health consultations through e-mail or telephone on evidence-based interventions to reduce disordered behaviors. Also, Tyler was placed on two different psychotropic medications on the basis of psycho-diagnostic tests and medical evaluation by his neurologist, his pediatrician, his play therapist, and his psychiatrist: Risperdal (Risperidone), an atypical antipsychotic; and Concerta (methylphenidate), a stimulant. Some of these psychotropic medications' side effects include difficulty falling asleep and remaining asleep throughout a night's cycle, decreased appetite, and anxiety.

Treatment

At the initial session, Tyler appeared to be a cheerful, energetic child who smiled frequently and seemed genuinely curious about the world. The therapist stated, "In here, you can play with all of the toys in most of the ways you want." From the very beginning of play therapy, Tyler seemed to be seeking a place or social relationship that would be stable. Perhaps Tyler felt safe and protected within the *temenos* of the playroom, a place where he was told that he would not be judged, a place where he would find 45 minutes of peace each week outside the tumultuous external reality he was experiencing. The therapist commented, "I've spoken to your mom, as she's told you, and I know that things have been difficult lately. I'm not sure how things will work out, as sometimes things don't always end happy, but I do know that I will be here with you." Tyler smiled and began his exploratory play.

During the first few sessions, Tyler engaged in exploratory play by examining the dollhouse, art supplies, sand tray, puppet house and puppets, sand figurines, and costumes in the drawers underneath the sand tray. His presentation indicated that he was coping with an extraordinary amount of anxiety because he would intermittently stop playing and bite his nails nervously. Afterward, he would smile and then frenetically shift to a different toy. He also had difficulty sitting still, staying focused on one task, and remembering things he had done in previous sessions. Strengths observed in his first few assessment sessions included his infectious energy and exuberance for life, his uncanny ability to listen and respond accordingly (when he wanted to), and his advanced verbal and reasoning skills. After manipulating the sand figurines and sand tray during the first three sessions, in the fourth session he asked the therapist, "What do kids do with this? Should I build a sand castle?" The play therapist responded, "In here, you can decide that. Some children create pictures in the sand. Maybe they place those figures (pointing to the sand figures) in the sand however they want and tell a story or show something. We usually call it *sandplay*." Tyler immediately began building his sand picture, and this led to the inception of the sandplay process.

At Tyler's first sandplay session, as well as in sessions 4 to 8, he repeatedly, chaotically tossed figures over his head and into the sand tray, peering at the play therapist and laughing playfully while he did this. There was a joy in him while he created these worlds, with figures piled on top of each other in a disorganized pattern with no discernible configuration. Chaos, usually characterized by a child's dumping several toys into the sand tray, not necessarily with form or foundation, may be symbolic of the child's ego being overwhelmed by distressing emotions (Allan, 1988).

The play therapist interpreted Tyler's sandplay as a mirroring of his emotional landscape, which was fraught with confusion, distraction, and destruction. As the play therapist observed these initial sand worlds of chaos, he empathized with Tyler's play and the affect he demonstrated while playing. The therapist felt a predominant sense of powerlessness and decimation in viewing Tyler's sand pictures once they were completed. This insight added to the clinical picture and gave the play therapist important affective information on which to rely when making interpretations. During session 8, after Tyler made another sand picture of chaos, the play therapist provided an interpretation after it was complete: "Tyler, when I watched you build this world, I felt like if I would be in it, it would be very scary. Nothing seems to go together or make much sense. I would probably hide underneath there (pointing to a bridge) to feel safe." It is interesting that Tyler replied, "Aw, if you felt scared, I would take care of you. Nothing bad would happen to you here." In this exchange, components of Tyler's good-enough parental projections were transferred to the play therapist.

In sessions 9 and 10, Tyler's sand pictures contained pandemonium, but the chaos was more organized and had structure. The Self had begun the process of constellating. For instance, Tyler began creating a picture with army men and epic battles with two red dragons. The army men were lined up, shooting the dragons. The dragons would breathe fire and incinerate a majority of the army. However, the story never contained a definitive ending; after the destruction, Tyler would throw different sand figurines into the sand tray and laugh mischievously. The play therapist asked, "What happened after the dragons destroyed the army?" Tyler replied, "I don't know," and continued tossing sand figurines into the sand tray. Here, his ego may have been coming to terms with the shadowy sides of his destructive temperament. Because it was so overwhelming, he discontinued the flow of the play to protect his ego. However, the play therapist viewed this as progress, because Tyler was beginning to tell his story symbolically through the sand scene. The play therapist was accepting of Tyler and his emotional pain.

During the first three months of play therapy, the play therapist conducted frequent mental health consultations with Tyler's teacher and school counselor. With the teacher, these consultations consisted primarily of cognitive behavioral interventions that she could implement to reduce disordered behaviors, and it also contained a bit of psycho-education on Oppositional Defiant Disorder and Attention-Deficit/Hyperactivity Disorder. With the school counselor, the play therapist coordinated services for Tyler to receive weekly problem-solving skills training in group counseling with male peers. Also, Charlotte participated in family play therapy sessions every two to three weeks. Infusing evidence-based interventions, the therapist augmented the traditional family play therapy paradigm with behaviorally oriented parent training. This included therapeutic limit setting, time-out, ignoring, parent praise, problem solving, psycho-education, and implementing tangible rewards (Chorpita et al., 2007).

During the week of session 9, the play therapist received this summary of Tyler's social progress from his preschool teacher during a consultation:

- showed care and concern for other's well-being,
- took responsibility for rules of the classroom,
- initiated consequences when he did not follow classroom rules,
- became liked by his male peers,
- enjoyed being the teacher's helper,
- greeted students every morning,
- told the teacher when he was upset or needed to talk,
- took his behavioral contract seriously,
- responded to warnings when given options, and
- decreased aggressiveness.

In sessions 11 to 16, Charlotte and Tyler's grandparents began commenting on the positive behavioral changes Tyler was exhibiting. However, Tyler's grandmother brought to the play therapist's attention that Tyler had been drawing some disturbing, dark images of monsters and talked about pain and death. The play therapist empathically responded and mentioned that sometimes when children are exorcising their demons in the playroom, darkness from the bottom of their psyches bubbles to the surface like crude oil from a well. This process, also called "the blackening" by alchemists (Moore, 2008), was tangibly represented by Tyler's raw material appearing in charred form. Just as alchemists burned elements and metals to ash to make gold, Tyler safely explored his inner darkness with the facilitation of a supportive therapist so that his self-healing (i.e., gold) could activate.

Tyler continued the theme of epic battles, but the battles became organized. The dragons continued to dominate the scenes, but the size of the army was augmented. The army men were delineated in military lineups with precision: the front lines contained cannons and the back rows of army men carried rifles for sniper fire. In the middle of the ferocious battle scene was a small bridge. Bridges may represent a child's transitional space, or connection, between the inner and outer worlds (Bradway & McCoard, 2005). After Tyler finished one of his epic battle scenes in session 15, he commented (in a loud voice), "The army men are tired of fighting and just want the dragons to leave them alone." The therapist, staying at the child's feeling level and within the metaphor, responded, "It sounds like the army is very brave but tired of fighting every day. Is there anything they could do to make the dragons leave them alone?"

Tyler thought about the therapist's question for a few seconds, then grabbed a green-colored jewel from the sand figures and placed it in the middle of the curve of the bridge. With a look of amazement (as though this was the first time he realized something could prevent the dragons from coming into the world), Tyler uttered in a triumphant tone, "This could do it. This is a magic jewel that makes the dragons sleep. And as long as the army keeps it on the bridge, the dragons will stay away." He became noticeably calm, and his affect regulated. The therapist reflected back the feeling and content: "The sand picture looks like it's finally at peace. Like maybe the army men are relieved because they aren't fighting the dragons all the time, even though everyone already knows that they are fearless. I noticed how the army can be brave warriors yet want peace. They have two opposite feelings at the same time, and that gives them strength and courage." Tyler replied, "I know. They are brave like me." Here, Tyler depicts his self-healing archetype as a green stone. Also, the army men were green in color, and he chose green construction paper for several art activities. According to Allan (1988), the color green may point to an escape from overwhelming anxiety, such when the green stone prohibited the destructive dragons from fighting with the army. Allan went on to say that green may represent "a sense of controlled behavior, a return to an untroubled nature" (p. 147).

During the time of sessions 17 to 20, Tyler began to exhibit marked improvements in behavior at home and at school. His mother, Charlotte, commented that he listened to directions at home, was less argumentative, was able to express his feelings when he was mad without hitting anything, and had not been in trouble at school for several weeks. Tyler's *Self* began to constellate the good-enough-parent imagoes and presented a shift in archetypal motifs in sandplay from destruction decay to nurturance compassion.

Termination

After eight months of coordinated multi-disciplinary services, including weekly play therapy sessions, Tyler demonstrated behavioral improvement and a cessation of many of the disruptive behaviors he had presented with at the inception of play therapy. To mark the occasion as celebratory, the play therapist held a "good-bye celebration," and cookies and punch were provided. For the first 30 minutes, Tyler and his play therapist reviewed the past eight months together in play and the good decisions Tyler was making. Tyler asked, "Are you proud of me?" The therapist smiled and responded, "What matters most is what you think. I, along with your family, care about you and whether or not you make good or bad choices. I am so pleased with all of the effort you have made to getting along with others. You did that!" Tyler responded, "OK. But are you proud of me for not being a bad boy anymore? That's what I wanna know!" The therapist responded in a gentle, caring tone, "You never were a bad boy. It's just that sometimes you made bad choices. And everyone does that sometimes, including me. What I've learned about you is that you deeply care for those around you and are working hard to show them without hurting them. You've been brave to try to make things different or better for you and your family." After hearing this encouragement, Tyler grinned. During the last 15 minutes, the play therapist invited Charlotte to join the good-bye celebration. The psychotherapy ended on a positive note of transitioning out of the safety and security of the playroom to the outer world, where Tyler had discovered the inner strength and familial and community support to resolve some of his emotional and behavioral difficulties.

4

Spontaneous Drawings

The aim of therapy is not acceptance, happiness, or adjustment. It's
a transparent, undefended heart.

—Thomas Moore

———

This chapter focuses on a case study involving a child and his family
who were traumatized and displaced by a natural disaster. While the
family stayed in a Red Cross shelter, the author used Jungian Play
Therapy with the child and the family, after Psychological First Aid
was administered, to help resolve some of the reactive symptoms
affiliated with Acute Stress Disorder. The self-healing archetype
emerged through the safe, trusting relationship between the child
and the therapist by means of an analytical attitude. The analytical
technique highlighted in this chapter is spontaneous drawings.

According to Baggerly and Green (2013), natural disasters are destructive events caused by nature that meet the following seven criteria: They
(1) cause destruction of property, injury, or loss of life, (2) have identifi-
able beginnings and ends, (3) are sudden and time-limited, (4) adversely
affect a large group of people, (5) are public events that affect more than
one family, (6) are outside the realm of ordinary experience, and (7) are psychologically traumatic enough to induce stress in almost anyone (Rosenfeld
et al., 2005). A destructive event is considered a "disaster" only when local
capacity and external resources have been overwhelmed. Likewise, the definition of disaster implies that the event causes psychological trauma that
would overwhelm the vulnerable child's ego. Just as first responders rush

to meet physical needs of overwhelmed survivors, so must Jungian play therapists facilitate the path of psychological healing in child trauma survivors. In a representative sample survey of 2,030 U.S. children ages 2 to 17, Becker-Blease, Turner, and Finkelhor (2010) found that approximately 14% reported a lifetime exposure to a disaster, and for 4.1% the event took place in the past year (Baggerly & Green, 2013).

Natural disasters can contribute to short-term and long-term disruptions in children's psychosocial, academic, and behavior functioning (Baggerly & Green, 2013). Black (2001) summarized the short- and long-term impact of natural disasters as follows: children who live through a disaster usually have two life-changing experiences. First, they endure the trauma itself, which might forever alter their sense of security and their ability to cope with life's problems. Second, they face ongoing disorder and dishevelment in their day-to-day lives (p. 54).

After a disaster, children ages 6 to 11 may exhibit typical reactions such as anxiety about family members' safety, fear that another disaster will occur, clinging or dependent behavior, bed-wetting, social withdrawal, increased fighting, hyperactivity, inattentiveness, irrational fears, irritability, sleep disruption, stomachaches, and school refusal (Baggerly & Green, 2013; Brymer et al., 2006; La Greca, 2008). In adolescents ages 12 to 18, common reactions include flashbacks and nightmares, emotional numbing, avoidance of reminders, substance abuse, depression, headaches and stomachaches, risk-taking behaviors, lack of concentration, apathy about school performance, and rebellion at home or at school (Brymer et al., 2006; La Greca, 2008). After disasters, both elementary and secondary school children who are displaced may have decreased school performance, including lower standardized test scores, tardiness, absenteeism, fights, verbal abuse of teachers, bullying, cutting class, and theft (Pane et al., 2008). Although these reactions to disasters typically resolve in most children within a short time, children may experience severe and ongoing symptoms such as depression, anxiety, and Post-Traumatic Stress Disorder (PTSD) for months and years if left untreated (Kronenberg et al., 2010).

Evidence-Based Approaches for Treatment

Evidence-based approaches for the prevention and treatment of severe symptoms in children affected by a disaster are selected based on the phase of disaster (La Greca & Silverman, 2009). The first phase of a disaster is pre-impact, at which time planning, training, and preparation is conducted before a disaster occurs. Evidence from La Greca and Silverman (2009) suggests that the most appropriate intervention during this phase is cognitive behavioral psycho-education to increase understanding of disasters and coping mechanisms in children and family members. The second phase is the impact phase, which occurs immediately after a disaster. La Greca and Silverman (2009) stated that the intervention with the most evidence is Psychological First Aid (PFA). "PFA is an evidence-informed modular approach to help children, adolescents, adults, and families . . . designed to reduce the initial distress caused by traumatic events and to foster short- and long-term adaptive functioning and coping" (Brymer et al., 2006, p. 5). This intervention is delivered one-on-one in about 15 to 20 minutes, usually at a disaster relief center, a medical facility, or near the site of the disaster after safety has been established.

The third phase of disaster recovery is short-term adaptation, which usually occurs days and weeks after a disaster (Baggerly & Green, 2013). One approach with strong evidence that has been used with children in fourth grade and above is cognitive behavioral interventions after trauma in schools (CBITS) (Jaycox et al., 2010). CBITS was designed to be delivered in 10 group sessions and one to three individual sessions in a school setting. After CBITS was provided to 57 fourth- through eighth-grade children with high trauma exposure during Hurricane Katrina and resulting clinical symptoms, these children showed clinically and statistically significant reduction in PTSD and depression (Jaycox et al., 2010).

The fourth phase of disaster recovery is long-term adaptation, which usually occurs months and years after the disaster. La Greca and Silverman (2009) stated that the intervention with the strongest evidence during this phase is trauma-focused cognitive behavioral therapy (TF-CBT) (Cohen et al., 2006). TF-CBT helps resolve trauma symptoms in children through strategies summarized in the acronym PRACTICE: Psycho-education and parenting skills, Relaxation, Affect modulation, Cognitive coping and processing, Trauma narrative, In vivo mastery of trauma reminders, Conjoint child-parent sessions, and Enhancing future safety and development. This is also the phase where it is most appropriate for highly trained and skilled play therapists to incorporate Jungian Play Therapy with children as well.

Landreth (2012) stated that the premise of play therapy is to use the therapeutic, nonjudgmental, permissive relationship between therapist and child to promote healing in children ages 3 through 10. Therapists utilize toys, art, sand, and other play media as the primary media for communication with clients. The evidence base for the effective practice of play therapy has grown in the new millennium (Baggerly et al., 2010). Bratton and colleagues' (2005) meta-analysis of 93 play therapy research studies demonstrated an effect size of .80, indicating a large treatment effect. There is also evidence that play therapy is an effective intervention for school children's academic achievement and their disaster recovery. After a large earthquake struck Taiwan, Shen (2002) demonstrated that child-centered play therapy (CCPT) significantly decreased children's anxiety and suicidal risk when compared to the control group.

In contrast to the nondirective approach of child-centered play therapy, many clinicians use a directive play therapy approach of cognitive behavioral play therapy (CBPT) (Knell & Dasari, 2009). CBPT is demonstrated as having a small to moderate treatment effect size when utilized with traumatized children (Drewes, 2009). Cognitive behavioral play therapy's premise is that cognitions shape behaviors and that the reconceptualization of distorted or faulty thinking or attributions of traumatic events by children will change their maladaptive behaviors and relieve anxieties. Young children's egocentric thinking may cause them to believe that they are solely responsible for problematic or disastrous occurrences. By utilizing therapeutic toys such as puppets or relaxation exercises, the school counselor educates students to promote understanding of the traumatic event and master coping behaviors.

In an effort to combine the child-directed approach of CCPT and the directive approach of CBPT, Gil (2011) developed trauma-focused integrative play therapy (T-FIPT) to provide post-traumatic treatment for children. T-FIPT integrates tenets of CCPT (e.g., nonjudgmental therapeutic relationships) and CBT strategies into play and expressive arts therapies. By using T-FIPT, therapists can provide the integrative work that respects the student's pacing, defensive mechanisms, and symbolic play as well as more directive interventions to assist the student's processing of trauma. Additionally, the T-FIPT model advocates for guardian/parental involvement in treatment as an effective adjunct to any type of traumatic treatment intervention. Although CBITS and TF-CBT have strong evidence for decreasing trauma symptoms after disasters, the author, as well as many leading clinicians in the disaster mental health field, recommends that therapists integrate play, PFA, CBITS, and TF-CBT as well as the expressive art therapy components of the visual approach within Jungian Play Therapy when they work with children traumatized by a disaster.

A Jungian Perspective on the Child's Inner World of Trauma

In this section, theoretical commentary is offered on the phenomenology of daimonic figures that appeared in many of the children's artwork and dreams following the author's disaster mental health work with children in Louisiana following Hurricanes Katrina and Rita as well as in Moore, Oklahoma, after the deadly tornadoes in 2013. Kalsched (1996) described the word *daimonic* as derived from *daioma,* which refers to division—breakthroughs or a divide between the conscious and the unconscious realm. Where significant trauma, such as separation or the intense disruption of the family system owing to mass destruction, has rendered psychic integration inoperable, children may dissociate (Jung, 1959). Dissociation is represented by the daimon that personifies the psyche's dissociative defenses (Kalsched, 1996). In dissociation, the child's psyche tricks itself into cutting off the harmful, unbearable external elements of the trauma and suppresses it to the unconscious, so the trauma becomes removed (or suppressed) from consciousness. For children who have experienced catastrophic devastation of their fragile egos (the center of consciousness, the "I" as we know ourselves), as happened to those who were rescued from life-threatening floods and saw dead bodies floating in putrid, stagnate water during Katrina, the psychological sequelae of the trauma become toxic to their interior life. Specifically, Jung (1963) stated that these trauma-induced complexes—strong images surrounded by gripping emotions—are represented in children's dreams and artwork by diabolical images (e.g., monsters, villains, dark figures, violence, death). For example, "Anthony," a 9-year-old boy who barely survived Katrina's flood waters, only to be tragically separated from his mother in a crowd, drew a series of images that contained variations of the same elements: water, a sinking ship, and a black shark fin placed ominously within the water (see "Case Illustration" in this chapter). All identifying information about clients presented in this chapter has been disguised.

When unimaginable anxiety overwhelms the child, as in catastrophic events or separation from primary caregivers during a natural disaster, the child's "transitional space" is severely compromised. According to Kalsched (1996), the "transitional space" is the realm between the inner and the outer worlds where the child learns how to play creatively and utilizes symbols. Severe traumatic anxiety effectively dismantles the "transitional space" and extinguishes the child's capacity to be creative through symbolic play, thereby inducing a fantasy state that is soothing and serves as a pathogenic anxiety-avoidance mechanism. This escape of fantasy and avoidance can become a pathological obsession for the child's conscious state, an auto-hypnotic twilight existence in which a delusive reality becomes the *only* reality. For example, Anthony repeatedly had dreams of an angel taking care of a baby, and he stated that the baby represented himself. Here, the good mother archetype appears in Anthony's dream to nurture the wounded child and relieve some of the psychic disintegration. Taking refuge at a Red Cross shelter, Anthony became fixated with playing video games that contained aggressive themes, and he neglected to eat and even defecated in his pants a couple of times because of his inability to recognize his somatic needs. Possibly, the video games depicted violent scenes that resonated with his own traumatic experience.

Children who are separated from or lose family members to death during a disaster suffer a *disconnect* to their ego's stability in managing the external world. Specifically, children affected by disasters often display an extremely poor connection with their unconscious. This is a result of the erosion of the "transitional space" between their outer and inner worlds because of the destabilization of their "good enough" parental introjects (images and the feelings associated with those images of the good mother or good father archetypes that provide safety). In order for the child's ego to resolve the decimating effects of trauma, a meaningful integration must occur. Meaning, according to Kalsched (1996), occurs when children's bodily excitations are given mental representation by transitional archetypal figures so that they eventually can reach verbal or symbolic expression and be shared with a trusting, caring individual. Helping a child recover the tenuous "transitional space," so that her creative capacities are restored, entails the enhancement of the connection between the unconscious and the conscious (Allan, 1993; Jung, 1963). From a Jungian perspective, this *coniunctio oppositorum*, or joining of opposites, portrayed in the child's drawing, painting, and/or verbalization of symbolic images (Furth, 1988) from dreams or the unconscious in the presence of a nonjudgmental, empathic therapist, facilitates psychological healing during extraordinary adversity (Allan, 1988; Green, 2005).

Serial Drawing: A Jungian Play Therapy Technique with Children Following Natural Disasters

Serial drawing is a therapeutic approach based on Jungian concepts that involves having a child produce drawings over time, thereby providing a view of the child's inner world to the therapist (Allan, 1988). After a therapeutic relationship and/or trust is formed between the therapist and the child, problems are expressed symbolically in the drawings, and healing and resolution of inner conflicts occur (Allan, 1988; Furth, 1988; Green, 2004). In the serial drawing technique, a therapist meets with a child regularly and asks him to "draw a picture while we talk." Jung (1963) believed that in times of significant crisis, children could turn inward toward the unconscious for dreams and images that carried within them the potential for healing—otherwise known as the self-healing archetype. From this perspective, the Jungian play therapist does not analyze the child's images but rather (a) encourages the child to make the images freely, with little to no direction from the therapist, (b) allows the child to absorb the image fully, so that the image can lead the child wherever she may need to go (toward self-healing), and (c) links the meaning of the symbols with the child's outer world at the point where the child's ego can accept and integrate the bridge between "transitional spaces." To reiterate, the serial drawing alone does not heal; rather, the self-healing archetype in children is activated by a curative alliance with a nonjudgmental therapist (Green, 2006). The serial drawing provides for a safe expression and exploration of feelings associated with the child's traumatic experience.

According to Walsh and Allan (1994), therapists may employ three different therapeutic styles when utilizing the serial drawing technique with children: (1) directive (the therapist gives the child specific images to draw, related to the trauma), (2) nondirective (the therapist simply says "draw whatever you'd like"), and (3) semi-directive (the therapist intermittently asks the child to redraw a specific symbol already produced, to further explore its inherently healing capacities). While individual children move at their own pace in self-healing, according to their developmental stage and also the nature of the trauma, general patterns in producing images in the serial drawing technique have been observed by Allan (2004). In the *initial stage* (typically the first few sessions), the drawings (a) provide a glimpse of the child's interior illustrated by symbols that reflect the source of trauma,

(b) reflect loss of internal or external control, with feelings of despair, and (c) establish initial rapport between the therapist and the child. In the *middle stage* (generally sessions 5–8), the child's drawings reflect (a) a pure expression of intense emotion, (b) struggles between conflicting internal polarities (loss of control versus mastery), and (c) the deepening of the therapeutic relationship between the child and the therapist, which is exemplified by the child talking directly about a traumatic issue or disclosing private and painful memories of the crisis to the therapist. In the *final stage* (sessions 9–12 and beyond), the child's drawings tend to depict (a) images that reflect a sense of mastery, self-control, and valuation, (b) scenes with positive imagery, (c) a depiction of the Self (intact self-portraits or mandalas [circular shapes connoting wholeness/integration]), (d) scenes that are humorous with no macabre references, and (e) artwork representing autonomy from the therapeutic relationship.

Not all children follow sequentially or pass through the aforementioned stages, and therapists should expect the unexpected when conducting serial drawings. In addition to a tolerance for ambiguity, therapists should provide an atmosphere that contains unconditional positive regard, trust, genuineness, warmth, and empathy, which may help children draw freely in a protected space (Hebert & Green, 2005). To process the serial drawing and amplify its symbols, Allan (2004) suggested that the therapist ask the child one or more of the following questions: (a) Does this picture tell a story? (b) I'm wondering if you can tell me what is happening in this scene? (c) If you could give this picture a title, what would it be? (d) If you were inside this picture, what would it feel like? (e) What went on in the story before this scene occurred? What happens next? (f) Could you tell me what you were thinking or feeling as you drew this? and (g) What does (identify a certain object or symbol in the picture) this mean to you?

During the processing of drawings, it is important for the therapist to remember that verbal and nonverbal communications to the child should reflect support, because in that way the child will come to realize that both good and horrible feelings are acceptable to convey in the therapeutic relationship. The next section demonstrates many of the Jungian principles outlined thus far in the chapter by describing a clinical vignette involving Jungian Play Therapy with a 9-year-old traumatized child separated from his primary caretaker during Hurricane Katrina, then later reunited with his family at a Red Cross shelter.

Case Illustration

This family consisted of the father, Gerry, in his mid-30s, unemployed; the mother, Belinda, in her early 30s, a secretary at an oil company; and the son, Anthony, age 9, in the fourth grade.

Presenting Problem

Almost immediately upon arrival at the Red Cross shelter in Lafayette, Louisiana, approximately two and a half weeks after Katrina made landfall east of New Orleans, I was approached by Gerry. A modest man with a low-pitched voice and a disheveled appearance, Gerry asked my assistance with helping his son, Anthony, and provided me with the following background information. Gerry, Belinda, and Anthony lived in an impoverished, dilapidated, crime-ridden section of New Orleans—the Ninth Ward. They did not have transportation and were unable to vacate the city when Mayor Nagin issued the mandatory evacuation order the night before Katrina came ashore. As Katrina's eye passed over New Orleans, their situation became precipitously dangerous. Specifically, the rising flood waters seeped into their living room through the home's front door. Riding out the storm overnight, they believed the worst was behind them. As the rain and wind continued to pummel the city into the next day, the levees were breached and the true horror began. Gerry described the rising waters as pouring into his home so fast that his family barely had time to climb into their attic. The floodwaters rose to the floor of the attic, completely inundating the house with water and debris. Without an escape route, the family remained stuck in the attic with no food or water for nearly 30 hours, hoping the floodwaters would recede. Eventually, Gerry used his rifle, which was stored in the attic, to blow several holes through the roof so he and his family could escape. The oppressive heat, combined with the humidity, reached sweltering heights as the family sat on the roof nearly eight hours in desperation. Finally, they were spotted and air-lifted to the New Orleans Convention Center. While there, Belinda was inadvertently separated from Gerry and her son in the mass hysteria of the crowd, which comprised thousands of angry, shocked, and terrified people. Luckily, Gerry and Anthony remained together and were bused to a shelter in Lafayette, Louisiana. Belinda was reunited with her family at the Red Cross shelter in Lafayette three days later.

After being separated from his mother, Anthony exhibited uncontrollable fits of crying and panic. When he was reunited with his mother at the shelter, Anthony did not appear relieved—instead he isolated himself. He spent several hours playing video games daily in the shelter. At night, Belinda said, he would wake up screaming periodically, waking others up, and then return to sleep—then not remember anything the next morning. Gerry asked if I would speak to his son, stating, "Anthony is like a different kid. It's like he's somebody else. He's very sad, and we don't know how to help him." I asked Gerry about Anthony's favorite activities, and he said they were drawing and playing soccer.

First Contact with the Child

My initial contact with Anthony occurred in the main room of the shelter following lunch. He was playing chess with his mother on her cot. Gerry introduced me to his son, and our first session began.

> *Gerry* (looking nervously at his wife): Belinda, I'd like you to meet Dr. Green. (Belinda smiles and immediately looks at her son.) Anthony, sit up, son, and introduce yourself to Dr. Green.
>
> *Anthony* (with a bewildered look on his face and looking right at me): I'm not sick. I don't need a doctor.
>
> *Dr. Green*: Hi Anthony. I'm sorry to interrupt your chess game. It looks like you were winning. You must be pretty good at chess huh? (Anthony smiles.) I'm not the kind of doctor that helps kids when they are sick. I'm the kind that helps kids when they have worries and maybe want to play and get their mind off of whatever is bothering them. I have an entire play area filled with toys and puppets. Why don't you come over and look at it, and see if you can find something you like. If you want, your mom and dad can come too.
>
> *Anthony*: Um. No thanks.
>
> *Dr. Green*: Ok. Well, just know that I'll be over there if you ever want look at the toys, and I even have a bunch of art supplies if you like to draw or paint.
>
> *Anthony*: You do? (He looks at his mom tacitly for permission. His mother nods her head agreeably and smiles.) Ok.

Anthony initially believed I was a medical doctor who had come to take care of the infirmed in the shelter. I began by trying to be polite and excusing myself for interrupting his chess game. Next, I gently clarified my purpose of being there so that Anthony did not feel embarrassed in any way in front of his parents for mistaking my profession. I gave him the choice to bring his parents with him because I wanted him to feel protected and safe, as I was a new face. Anthony was not all that interested in leaving his mom to go off with me to see a play area. I did not view this as resistance but as progress toward developing rapport. Feeling like we had made progress just by talking, I left with an open invitation to draw, an activity Anthony enjoyed, and he accepted.

After exploring the play area over a period of approximately 10 minutes, Anthony thanked me for inviting him and walked back to his parents. As he was leaving, I stated that if he wanted to come back later he could, since I would be there in the mornings and evenings. Anthony did come back the next morning, and he participated in eight play therapy sessions with me over the course of eight consecutive days. After the eighth day, he and his family were relocated to another shelter.

Preliminary Assessment and Treatment Plan

Upon my initial contact and observations with Anthony, and also my communications with his parents, it appeared that Anthony was responding to the overwhelming stimuli of his traumatic experience by socially withdrawing, perhaps providing his psyche time to heal from the state of overstimulation. In the course of two weeks, Anthony had been trapped in rising floodwaters, had gone without food or water for almost two days in squalid, blisteringly hot conditions, had witnessed his home flooded and destroyed, and had been separated from his mother during a chaotic scene at an overpopulated refuge center. He was now living in a large open room inside a shelter with people he did not know. All of these external events would appear to have been able to overwhelm the fragile ego of any child (or even any adult), but Anthony seemed remarkably resilient. While he appeared to be in good health, his compulsive video-game playing for hours at a time without speaking to anyone, his social isolation and dysphoric demeanor, and his soiling himself were signs that he was suffering from traumatic stress-related symptoms. Because of the transient nature of the shelter and the limited scope of crisis intervention counseling, I set up a basic, simple treatment plan for Anthony:

- Provide Anthony a safe, grounded space where he could relax and feel open to share his feelings either verbally or symbolically
- Strengthen Anthony's ego so that he could bolster his coping skills
- Reduce Anthony's anxiety (e.g., nightmares and midnight screams, which were waking up those around him in the shelter) by allowing his unconscious to be represented in the play area, where he could begin to regain mastery of his feelings

Anthony enjoyed drawing and painting; therefore my aim was to sit quietly and allow him to create whatever he wanted. By the time I met Anthony, which was roughly two weeks after he had entered the shelter, he had discontinued some of his behavioral manifestations of trauma and was mainly having difficulties coping and expressing his emotions. Because of the time frame of trauma, I chose to utilize both nondirective and some semi-directive techniques. Shen (2002) stated that nondirective approaches might work well with children affected by trauma who are no longer exhibiting reactive symptoms but who are having coping difficulties. Utilizing a Jungian Play Therapy framework that combines nondirective and directive approaches, the therapist must accept three premises when counseling children affected by trauma:

- Each child has an unconscious psyche, and if provided with a supportive and nonthreatening environment (or therapeutic "container"), it will reveal itself symbolically through spontaneous drawings, play, or dream content.
- Though play, drawings, and dreams are not direct forms of communication with a child, they are valid and have meaning. They give the therapist a glimpse into the child's internal struggles.
- The mind and the body are linked together, thereby allowing continuous communication between the two spheres, so that if something is troubling a child psychically, the body will communicate this, and vice-versa (Allan, 1988).

Segments/Summary of Play Therapy Sessions

The play therapy sessions began approximately two weeks after Anthony and his family entered the Red Cross shelter. Four of the play therapy sessions that occurred between Anthony and me took place in a makeshift play area (a storage room next to the kitchen area) inside the Red Cross shelter; the other four were completed outside the shelter at a picnic table near a lush green and wooded forestlike area.

SESSIONS 1–2

The first couple of sessions consisted of building rapport with Anthony, which proved to be easy. For all of his parent's concerns and reports of his maladaptive behaviors, he appeared to be adjusting as each day passed.

Upon entering the play area, I said to him, "Anthony, this is your play area while we are together. You can do most anything you want in here, except for hurting me or yourself. I'm just going to sit right here for now. When the big hand on the clock reaches the twelve, our time will be finished." After I finished with my initial introduction, Anthony moved directly toward the art supplies, which consisted of plain white paper and sharpened colored pencils. Creative artwork with materials such as paper, colored pencils, glue, and paints allows children to create freely what is going on in their lives (Furth, 1988) and comfortably express themselves within the therapeutic dyad. Allan (2004) suggested that white paper be utilized in the playroom to provide the children with a blank area on which to display their intrapsychic projections. As Anthony drew, I remained relatively quiet, not wanting to take the focus off of his artistic creation. During play sessions, while the child is drawing, the therapist sits near or beside the child. The therapist does not talk much in the beginning stages unless the child initiates conversation. The therapist does not initiate conversation or take any notes, but observes the child, how the child approaches the drawing, the placement of figures, and the types of images, symbols, and themes that emerge in the child's pictures (Allan, 1988).

In each of the first two sessions, Anthony spent approximately 15–25 minutes drawing a scene, and the two drawings looked very similar. The paper was largely covered by blue water, and within the water was a small ship that appeared to be broken in half. There was also a small dark shark fin in the water and a bright yellow sun at the top of the paper. In the first session, I asked him if he could describe to me what it would be like if he was on the boat in the scene. He said, "It would be scary 'cause it's sinking and everyone's 'gonna die." This scene provided me with a view of Anthony's internal world, containing themes of devastation and disaster. His response to the artwork and his affect while drawing seemed intense, reflecting the trauma's effect on Anthony's sense of stability and groundedness.

During the second session, when Anthony drew nearly exactly the same scene, the black shark fin was larger and the sun had rays beaming from it, whereas in the first picture the shark fin was relatively small and the sun was a simple yellow circle filled in with an orange color. In an effort to amplify the symbols, I asked Anthony if there was any way the people in the boat could find a life raft or save themselves in any way, and he responded, "No, the shark is going to eat them, and they will die in the water." With all of this macabre imagery, I noticed a bright, shining sun at the top of the scene. Anthony was possibly struggling with ambivalent feelings, so I watched him as he reflected on the image, absorbing its beauty; then I placed the drawing in my file and he left. Only after day 2 did I realize that the sun might be a source of healing for Anthony. I remembered that his father had said he enjoyed playing soccer outdoors, and now this sun symbol appeared in his artwork. Perhaps this could be his self-healing archetype, but I would not know until Anthony knew for himself.

SESSION 3

In the third play therapy session, Anthony again drew a scene similar to the first two drawings, this time with some interesting changes (fig. 4.1).

> *Dr. G*: A., You've really put a lot of effort into this scene. I am impressed (Anthony looks up at me for a second and smiles, then redirects his attention to the scene). I'm wondering if you could describe the scene to me.
>
> *A*: Well, It's these people that are trying to get away from this shark (pointing to the shark fin). And the shark is trying to kill them, and he's fast. The boat is trying to get away. But they're almost at the beach so the shark can't get them there.
>
> *Dr. G*: Ah, I see. I noticed in this picture that the boat is not broken in half or sinking like it was in the other scenes you drew. Do you know what made the boat be able to get away from the shark this time?
>
> *A* (thinks for a minute and murmurs "hmm" under his breath as if contemplating): It's because the sun was out and the wind was blowing and the sail just could go faster. That's it.
>
> *Dr. G*: Ok Anthony. Thank you for sharing your artwork with me. If you could give a name to this picture, what might it be called?
>
> *A* (without a second's hesitation): "The Flood."

Here, I was not praising Anthony, but encouraging his efforts. By asking him if he could describe the scene, I was attempting to get an understanding of what he was trying to convey, and I also helped him verbalize it so he could make the connections between his inner and outer worlds. In the scene, the boat is not broken in half, but intact. Also, Anthony added sand at the bottom, which was not present in the first two scenes. The shark fin has shrunk slightly in size from the previous scene. I got the sense while Anthony was talking that he was proud of his scene and in some way relieved

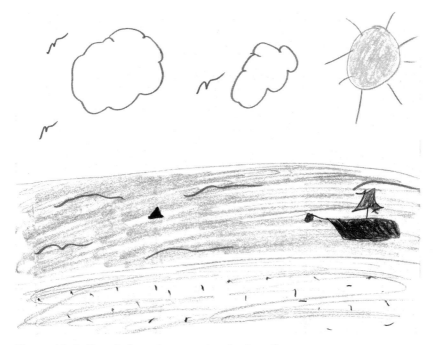

Figure 4.1. Anthony's "spontaneous drawing" no. 3

that the boat was outrunning the shark to shore. Additionally, he identified the sun and wind as protective forces in the picture that enabled the ship to get away from the shark. Finally, the title was important, because water was a recurring theme in Anthony's artwork, and also water was what nearly killed Anthony and his family when they were trapped in their attic. Through this artwork, his unconscious was attempting to make meaning out of the water and its devastating effects.

Anthony's drawing seemed to reflect Anthony's slow progress toward psychic integration of the trauma. Specifically, the presence of brown sand, or Earth, is a grounding feature of his third art scene. He commented that the boat is almost at the beach, where it is safe and the evil force—the shark—cannot harm the boat. And the sun is again present in this third scene, but this time it is more pronounced than in the other two scenes. In children's drawings, the sun can represent a healer, restorer, or a provider of warmth and understanding for development (Allan, 1988; Furth, 1988). The ocean or water typifies primordial waters, which are one of the four elements responsible for sustaining life. In a child's drawings, water can represent life and death, or it can illustrate the vast, formless unconscious of the child's nascent ego attempting to regenerate. Anthony's drawing in our third play therapy session seemed to reflect the activation of the self-healing archetype—the sun shone brightly and guided the boat to shore, where safety awaited from the dangerous shark. In other words, Anthony's transference onto me was beginning to activate his feelings of self-acceptance and caring, which created new psychological maturation.

SESSIONS 4–8

For the fourth session, I asked Anthony if he would enjoy going outside in the sunlight to draw. He excitedly agreed, and I accompanied him to gain permission from his mother. The reasoning for this change in location was that I wanted Anthony to be able to reconnect to nature in some way—with the sun and greenery—in an attempt to continue his psychological self-healing. Nature was helping the boat in his artwork escape from danger. As stated earlier, the Jungian play therapist believes in the mind-body connection. Therefore, I viewed the series of images as Anthony's mind telling his body to reconnect to the outdoors with fresh air, sunlight, and the Earth. Interestingly enough, Anthony's mother commented, "You know son, you haven't been going outside much at all lately. You love to play outside. Go have fun."

During the fourth play session, Anthony and I sat at a picnic table—located adjacent to the shelter, among many large trees and a small forested area—and he drew another scene. This scene was basically the same scene as before, except this time the boat was located at the shoreline. Also, people appeared in this scene, all of whom were positioned in the sand. This scene contained a dark shark fin protruding from the water, as in the last few scenes. After he finished, I asked him how he felt as he was drawing. Anthony replied, "I don't know. I felt sad, but kind of happy. . . . I was sad 'cause I almost drowned in some water like these people in the boat, except there was no shark, just water and maybe an alligator. But I'm happy 'cause I like the beach, and I wish we had a boat so we could have gotten away from the bad storm." Here, Anthony is disclosing deep issues and fears as he begins to trust more in me and the therapeutic relationship. This is the first time he has mentioned anything about his experience with Hurricane Katrina to me. With acceptance, I simply smiled and nodded my head to let him know I supported him and was there for him. This drawing seemed to reflect competency and coping, as the people in the boat made it to shore and were on the beach. The sun was present in this scene, a yellow mandala, which reflected the overall internalization of positive images. Later that afternoon, Belinda said that Anthony did not wake up screaming in the middle of the night. I asked her if she noticed any other changes, and she said, "No, not really. Well, maybe he's talking more now, but I don't know if that's what you mean." Anthony was slowing emerging from his self-imposed exile.

The fifth session occurred back in the play area and consisted of Anthony placing his crayons in a circular shape, a mandala, on the floor (fig. 4.2). From a Jungian perspective, when children draw or create mandalas, it is representative of some type of psychic healing—the child's internal striving toward wholeness. According to Allan (2004), mandalas represent the Self in union with the ego. The circle represents the ego's boundaries but refers to the Self at the same time in a state of congruence. Children's mandalas reflect the development of protective walls that function as an intrapsychic means of preventing psychological disintegration.

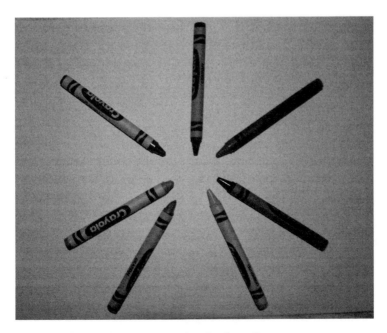

Figure 4.2. Anthony's "spontaneous drawing" no. 5

Without any probing, Anthony began to describe losing his mother at the convention center amid the chaos of people. As he told me his story, I listened and did not interrupt or ask any clarifying questions. He talked about being terribly frightened; surprisingly, he explained that his fears were more about his mother's safety and personal well-being than a fear of her not being there to meet his own emotional needs. Anthony was ready to share his pain with me, and it was my responsibility in that moment to simply "meet him where he was" in the pain. After this session ended, we returned inside the shelter; and he ran to his mother and hugged her. I smiled and walked back to the play area to begin another session with a different child.

Our sixth through eighth play sessions were all conducted outside with Anthony playing with a soccer ball while I mostly watched and tracked his play. He did not discuss his experiences during Katrina again. Anthony and his family were transferred to a shelter in a different city the day after our eighth session. Before they left, Anthony's mother gave me a hug, and Gerry and Anthony both shook my hand, with Anthony smiling, looking reticent to leave the shelter he had come to know as home for the past few weeks. I returned all of Anthony's artwork to him, and I directed him to think about the sun in his pictures when he was not feeling so good. He said, "Thank you," and they left.

Conclusion

Throughout our brief time together, I believed in Anthony's psyche's ability to heal itself. We began play therapy by going "into the wounding" and ended with him initiating curative strategies to heal himself. The life-threatening disaster and subsequent separation from his primary caregiver caused Anthony's de-integration of the Self and fragmentation of his fragile ego. However, the therapeutic relationship engendered a sense of safety for Anthony to express his feelings and allow his unconscious to be represented and connected to his conscious. As he created and embraced the symbols, they transformed into affect. Instead of unconsciously repressing the haunting images and feelings associated with the trauma, Anthony's ego began assimilating the trauma by painting its image in symbolic form (i.e., the sinking ship hunted by the shark). By acknowledging the feeling and the image, Anthony was able to change his affect. The archetype of the *Self* guided Anthony where he needed to go for the healing to activate.

For Jungian Play Therapy to be considered effective, the therapist must change just as much as the child. Both will influence each other: humanness is the critical point. Involvement of the therapist occurs on a continuum from active to passive, which influences the impact of therapy. Jungians might join in play, or accompany the child in his symbols and archetypal struggles in the underworld. Jungians possess a freedom to move along the therapeutic continuum by following the child and creating a safe space for the child's Self to evolve. In the clinical vignette involving Anthony, I found myself utterly struck by his resiliency and the power of his ego to re-constellate in the middle of such turmoil and psychic upheaval. As his ego became stronger, Anthony's behavioral impulses became less pronounced (i.e., his fixation with video games decreased, and his screaming in the middle of the night stopped).

Just as Anthony began to develop the skills to cope with the outside world, I noticed a transformation in my own coping style. I had experienced inherent trepidation about pushing children too far or not doing enough in disaster mental health work, and this fear, at times, consumed me. I coped with this fear by being hypervigilant and eschewing my inner guide. After I counseled Anthony, my coping style changed because I realized just how powerful the child's Self is for inner healing, and how little I needed to do. The symbols led brave Anthony toward his own inner healing. Therefore, I no longer maintained the heightened level of psycho-arousal and trusted more in the process. Just as the alchemists attempted to transmute lead into gold, I noticed a calming within me that converted my irrational fears of inadequacy into a modest self-assurance. I believe this had a positive effect on children in that the process of therapy seemed to flow more naturally from then on.

5

Expressive Arts

People say that what we're all seeking is a meaning for life. I don't think that's what we're really seeking. I think that what we're seeking is an experience of being alive, so that our life experiences on the purely physical plane will have resonances within our own innermost being and reality, so that we actually feel the rapture of being alive. That's what it's all finally about, and that's what these clues help us to find within ourselves.

—Joseph Campbell, *The Power of Myth*

The use of expressive arts with adolescents in play therapy is a creative, multi-modal treatment design that strengthens attachment. In a Jungian approach, a play therapist incorporates and honors the adolescent's symbols, images, sandplay pictures, and emotional containment throughout the clinical process. As new relationships develop and alter or dissipate over time, adolescents may experience variations and fluctuations in their mental well-being (Berger et al., 2005). Current research in parent-adolescent attachment relationships has demonstrated associations between secure, positive attachment and (a) lower mental health difficulties (Van Doorn et al., 2011), (b) meaningful relationships (McGee et al., 2006), and (c) increased career success (Shelton & van den Bree, 2010). This chapter provides a brief overview of the most current research in the area of adolescent attachment within the context of Jungian play psychotherapy, as well as clinical implications for incorporating Jungian play-based interventions, such as sandplay (Donald,

2003), in the consulting room with adolescents to increase attachment and feelings of psychological security.

Jungian Play Therapy (JPT) offers a less threatening alternative to traditional talk therapy between mental health clinicians and adolescents. JPT with adolescents is a particular form of play therapy, or *activity therapy*, that facilitates healing through the relationship and the externalization of images, metaphors, and symbols. The language of JPT is typically visual rather than verbal; Jungian play therapists encourage adolescents to produce and resonate with symbols through sandplay, art journals, guided imagery, dream work, and coloring mandalas. JTP can be a useful treatment approach because adolescents learn primarily through social observation, modeling, and reinforcement, which are facilitated by their relationships. Adolescent learners have innate preferences for either visual, auditory, kinesthetic, or haptic modalities when receiving new information. They have a proclivity for either concrete-sensory or abstract-intuitive thought; they sort what they know in creative random clusters or in a linear step-by-step sequence (Green, Schweiker, et al., 2009). JPT meets adolescents where they are developmentally by utilizing the crux of change, the therapeutic relationship, to engender a warm, supportive environment that induces a climate permeated by the safe expression of imagery and emotion.

The Mental Health Context of Developing Adolescents

Adolescents prefer either focused attention, acts of helpful service, physical affection, tangible gifts, or words of affirmation within relationships they label as helpful (Green, Schweiker, et al., 2009). A "one size fits all" approach to relating and counseling is ineffective with adolescents. They may initially present as docile, guarded, suspicious, or aggressive when starting psychotherapy. It is the responsibility of the therapist to forge an honest and caring relationship with the adolescent, mostly by imbuing genuineness and acceptance, if the therapeutic relationship is to emerge. Adolescents typically do not care what a therapist knows until they know that the therapist truly cares about them. A therapist must genuinely like adolescents and compassionately relate to the adolescents' psychosocial struggles, because the effectiveness of the counseling process depends upon it. When working with a teenager, a play therapist must typically utilize a strength-based approach. An adolescent may ignore the therapist as soon as gratuitous compliments or unwelcome advice are given (Green, Schweiker, et al., 2009). Adolescents typically see through the facade of uneasy adults. Moreover, they cannot be expected to resolve their interpersonal deficits if the adults who help them cannot acknowledge their own.

Creative, therapeutic activities provide the adolescent with emotional outlets, while decreasing the stigma associated with appearing socially awkward by talking to an older, unknown adult about their problems. For example, adolescents with externalizing behavioral problems are in conflict with others and themselves (Green, Schweiker, et al., 2009). The expressive art techniques associated with JPT may extend the emotional safety and freedom to explore who they are (identity), what they are doing (motivation), and the hidden emotions involved (affect). The analytical attitude of the therapist permits the adolescent to move from impulse or action to the symbolic life, where emotions and images are contained. By containing rage, therapists facilitate adolescents' transformative process, sublimating aggression into assertiveness, which typically brings forth positive feelings. Through the safety of the therapeutic dyad, aggression moves into assertiveness to help adolescents articulate and strategize their despair or self-inflicted alienation as opposed to nontherapeutically dwelling upon it.

The Therapeutic Relationship as the Centerpiece for Change

The play therapist's role in the therapeutic relationship with an adolescent is as observer-participant, using directive techniques that harness the adolescent's creativity in spontaneous drawings, drama play, or sandplay to bolster available ego-energies (Green, 2009a). Jungian therapists utilize art interpretation and analysis of transference to assess the archetypal or symbolic complex the adolescent is operating within, which often contains polarities. A *complex* is an unconscious assortment of strongly identified emotions or beliefs that influence behaviors. Jung believed that complexes may have been related to traumatic experiences. For example, the shadow was a primary complex in trauma (or ordinarily health) and was considered pathological depending on the evidence of destructive behaviors associated with the shadow. Jung's *shadow* is any aspect of the psyche that has been excluded from conscious awareness. Therefore, play therapists facilitate adolescents' discovery and integration of the dark side of their personality, the shadow, in an effort to maintain psychic equilibrium and promote psychological health.

Jungian play therapists counseling adolescents (a) make sense of symbols through an extensive process of personal work with a Jungian analyst; (b) conceptualize rage within an analytical framework (i.e., a broken attachment turns into rage and, if not remedied, depression and ultimately withdrawal); (c) maintain an *analytical attitude* that is both involved and detached; (d) possess the ability to direct adolescents' raw material by carrying some of their *psychological poison;* and (e) use sandplay, artwork, and dream analysis to amplify symbols and follow the adolescent's Self wherever it leads along the path to individuation. JPT with adolescents helps make connections between their difficult emotions, rigid defenses, and problematic behaviors through the acceptance, over time, of the symbols produced. The expressive arts within JPT identify difficult behaviors and how others perceive those behaviors and attitudes. In sandplay, adolescents may develop self-soothing and coping strategies.

Analytical Strategies with Adolescents

First, the play therapist and the adolescent must *surrender* the demands of the ego and formulate rapport built upon a trusting, emotionally safe (i.e., nonthreatening and nonjudgmental) therapeutic alliance (Green, 2009b). It is important for the play therapist to attend to subtle interactions in the analytical relationship while simultaneously engendering an emotional holding environment where the adolescent's ego feels safe to reveal itself. A second specific strategy is the *analysis of the transference.* Transference, within a Jungian framework, is not solely projections of the adolescent's personal past (e.g., parent complexes) onto the therapist, but also archetypal or nonpersonal projections the adolescent unwittingly transfers onto the therapist. The central aim of analyzing the transference is not to figure out what destructive forces led the adolescent to therapy, but to repair what's happening in the present moment through the therapeutic relationship. Dissimilar from Freud, Jung emphasized the importance of current conflicts created in the transference as more important than the interpretation and analysis of the adolescent's past infantile rage or pathology (Jung, 1964). Jungians not only acknowledge the problems that happened in the adolescent's past; they also acknowledge that these problems are healed in the present moment. This occurs through the *corrective emotional experience* inherent within the therapeutic relationship.

A third strategy used with adolescents is *amplification of symbols.* Jungian play therapists amplify symbols contained within the play or activity-based therapy, which means they make them more conscious both verbally and nonverbally through playful and creative interventions. Often, active imagination is used to facilitate the production of inner symbols so that the Self may lead the adolescent toward healing. Jung's definition of a symbol implies that it in itself is not able to be portrayed; rather, a symbol is the totality whose manifestations can be observed in the joining of the psyche's elements. All of these techniques and building a warm relationship lead to the central focus of adolescent play therapy: strengthening attachment.

Psychosocial Determinants and Effects of Divergent Attachments in Adolescents

Attachment is a dynamic pattern of cognitions, affect, and associated behaviors that result from a caregiver's ability to meet infants' need for warmth, nurturance, and safe physical closeness (Berger et al., 2005). Early in life, children develop an *internal working model* through their relationships with caregivers. This model incorporates the belief that either (1) one is worthy of love and the world is a predictable and positive place (i.e., *secure attachment*) or (2) one is unlovable and exists in a world that is unpredictable and untrustworthy (i.e., *insecure attachment*) (Bowlby, 1982). Secure and insecure attachments encompass ideas related to the idea that parents are able to tolerate or not tolerate, or contain, their child's intense emotional experiences until the child manages the experiences herself (Black et al., 2010; Briggs, 2003). *Disorganized attachment* (Main & Solomon, 1990) is demonstrated by a child who exhibits patterns of (a) clear avoidance (or resistance) in the first reunion and then a change to clear resistance (or avoidance) in the second reunion with the caretaker(s) or (b) evidence of sequential, contradictory behavior across separation and reunion episodes. This style of broken attachment typically stems from experiencing consistent frightening and comforting messages simultaneously from the caretaker(s), usually resulting from trauma (Green et al., 2010).

Although they tend to move toward confiding in peers as they move through puberty, many teenagers consider their parents primary supports and confidants (Nomaguchi, 2008). Some adolescents continue to rely on their parents throughout development; feeling secure in the parent-teen relationship allows them to embrace their curiosity about the world (Duchesne & Larose, 2007). Those adolescents who fear that their parents will not consistently provide a secure base are more likely to fear exploration, uncertainty, and/or vulnerability (Perl, 2008).

The Influence of Attachment on Adolescents' Psychology

Secure and insecure attachments have been linked with a number of psychosocial outcomes across the lifespan (Van Doorn et al., 2011), including those present in the cases of Nichole and Ilene that are highlighted later in this chapter. Attachment is thought to play a role in the development and maintenance of *internalizing symptoms,* such as anxiety and depression. Anxiety about peers and academic success, for example, is commonly reported in both clinical and nonclinical populations of adolescents (Gren-Landell et al., 2009). Theorists have suggested that closeness and trust within a secure parent-teen relationship may buffer against mood and anxiety symptoms by providing feelings of closeness and trust. Supporting research has demonstrated that as quality of attachment decreases, internalizing symptoms increase, and vice versa (Buist et al., 2004; Liu, 2007, 2008). However, the same process does not obtain in adolescents who predominantly externalize.

Parents who respond to their teens only in times of crisis or as a result of dangerous behavior put their teens in a situation where they must aggressively force their parents to meet their needs (van der Vorst et al., 2006). In accordance with this idea, high externalizing behaviors have been associated with low perceived attachment (Buist et al., 2004; Howard & Medway, 2004), anger and hostility (Muris et al., 2004; Simons et al., 2001) and early substance use (Hahm et al., 2003; Shelton & van den Bree, 2010; Steinberg, 2007). Furthermore, rates of *externalizing behaviors* increase drastically during adolescence and can include experimentation with drugs and alcohol, self-injurious behavior, and conflict in relationships. Some of the attachment literature demonstrates that adolescents partake in high-risk behaviors and, as noted in the next paragraph, nonsuicidal self-injurious behaviors, in an effort to engage the parent in caregiving behaviors (Steinberg, 2007).

Researchers have found that although parental relationships are still viewed favorably by many adolescents (Berger et al., 2005), peer relationships have a stronger influence over adolescents' emotional stability, psychological health, feelings of inclusiveness, and confidence (Hay & Ashman, 2003). As adolescence progresses, the significant and influence of peer friendships yield to burgeoning romantic relationships (Furman & Wehner, 1997), in which attachment style also plays a crucial role. Research on attachment and adolescent romantic relationships has demonstrated associations between insecure attachment and greater reported relationship stress (Seiffge-Krenke, 2006) and physical violence (Henderson et al., 2005), with some research having noted the increased potential for intimate partner violence when both parents demonstrate insecure attachment (Orcutt et al., 2005). These findings can be interpreted in several ways. One interpretation is that the degree of security in parental connections influences the degree of security in future social connections. Another is that the lack of a secure parental base from which to explore leaves the adolescent susceptible to engaging in psychologically unhealthy or "toxic" relationships. Still another is possibly that those with unstable relationships are not capable of providing the security desired (Furman et al., 2002).

Finally, adolescents' ability to successfully leave their parents' home, explore their independence, and partially support themselves or become completely autonomous following high school is largely grounded in the tenets of attachment theory (i.e., secure base, proximity, and safe haven): this has important implications in Western culture, where such autonomy is valued and encouraged. Moreover, adolescent-supported educational and career changes and decisions can be of significant distress especially if parental support and resources are at a minimum (Gaffner & Hazler, 2002; Multon et al., 2001). Adolescents who are insecurely attached to their caretakers may struggle to achieve balance between interpersonal relationships and autonomy, whereas adolescents who are securely attached possess the confidence that relationships will remain secure even as new life paths are navigated. Further, attachment security affects how well adolescents utilize significant adults in their lives to assist them in managing stress as new experiences present themselves (Larose & Boivin, 1998), with insecurely attached adolescents at risk for greater feelings of loneliness, anxiety, and stress (Vignoli et al., 2005) and inhibited environmental exploration (Green, Schweiker, et al., 2009) as compared to their securely attached counterparts.

The next section of the chapter comprises the biographical and psychosocial data of two adolescents in play therapy who struggled with insecure or broken attachments. The cases highlight how their path to healing was facilitated by the use of the therapeutic relationship as an analog to secure attachment. Moreover, sandplay and other expressive arts were used to strengthen attachment in the adolescents with their caretakers. All names in the case examples are pseudonyms, and some details have been altered to protect the clients' confidentiality.

Psychosocial Data and Attachment Considerations: Two Adolescent Case Illustrations

Ilene

Ilene was a 17-year-old female who came to treatment because of symptoms consistent with generalized anxiety and obsessive compulsive disorders. Examples of her symptoms included intense worries about academic performance, intricate compulsions related to concerns about safety, and poor sleep. Ilene had many friends, although she denied having a "best friend." Recently, she had become single after a romantic partner abruptly ended their relationship, and she described her relationships with her parents as "acceptable." She complained that everyone in her life expected her to be perfect and that she felt tremendous pressure to meet these unrealistic expectations. Ilene attended school consistently and received average grades. Moreover, she reported that of all of the people in her life, she felt most supported by members of the teaching staff at her high school. During her intake appointment, both parents highlighted Ilene's talents, her social involvement, and her physical attractiveness. They minimized her psychopathological symptoms and their impact on her psychosocial functioning, as well as their relationships with her. The father reported that Ilene believed his father-daughter relationship with her was less important than those with her peers. Ilene's mother discussed several failed attempts to improve the mother-daughter relationship.

As the alliance between the therapist and Ilene grew, Ilene's willingness to share increased. During one particularly difficult session, Ilene noted, "It's like I know you won't hate me or tell me not to come back if you know that I am not perfect." During this time, Ilene engaged in regular sandplay sessions, where she created pictures in a sand tray with miniatures, with no therapist-led direction before, during, or after. Ilene revealed that she felt neglected in her family and believed that her parents favored her older and younger sisters. She commented that her parents expected her to be independent and were reluctant to assist her when she requested their help; she also reported that they minimized her symptoms, calling them "silly" or "just for attention." According to Ilene, her mother regularly threatened to stop paying for her play therapy treatment, although her mother denied this when the play therapist brought the issue up during a private parent consult. Ilene reported that attempts to engage in family events or emphasize the importance of reliance on one another through family dinners and meetings were repeatedly rejected by both parents. Ilene repeatedly attempted to verbalize her feelings and thoughts to her father during family therapy sessions, but she reported to the play therapist that these attempts did not translate into any lasting changes after leaving the session.

Approximately six months into treatment, Ilene began considering colleges she might like to attend. Ilene told her play therapist that she vacillated between wanting to go "far, far away from [her] family" and worrying that her parents would forget about her if she went too far. On more than one occasion, she expressed innate and what she perceived as irrational fears about the anxiety surrounding attending a distant college and stopping therapy. She decided to apply to both local and distant colleges, with her first choice being a college that was approximately 120 miles from home.

Nichole

Nichole was a 14-year-old female who came to therapy because of depressive symptomatology and intermittent self-injurious behaviors. Nichole's parents were divorced, and her father reported a long-standing mental health history, including anxiety and Bipolar Disorder. Nichole's mother denied any mental health history, but she acknowledged that Nichole's two sisters and one brother had also struggled with anxious and depressive symptoms throughout their adolescence and early adult lives. Nichole described herself as "always trying to hide who I am" and as someone who regularly sacrificed her own happiness for that of her family members. She described this dynamic as being particularly evident in her relationship with her father, who had difficulty conversing with his daughter in meaningful ways. Nichole described her relationship with her mother as emotionally distant and strained, but it was one that she emotionally relied upon during difficult transitions. Nichole described herself as an "outsider" in her family.

Early in treatment, Nichole shared that she had recently become close with a male peer, Cordell, who was one year older than she. She believed that Cordell understood her and was accepting of her even when she was unhappy. This relationship progressed into a romantic one, and Nichole initially reported feeling a sense of happiness during their time together.

Within a few sessions, however, Nichole began reporting that Cordell became verbally abusive and controlling. She reported that he engaged in various manipulative and noxious behaviors, including these: (1) Cordell became angry if she ended a phone call with him when he was not ready for it to end, (2) Cordell became possessive of her free time during the weekend, so that she felt guilty about seeing anyone else, and (3) Cordell expressed disdain when she wanted to spend time with others. On more than one occasion, she claimed that he threatened to harm himself if she did not comply with his requests. Nichole kept the romantic nature of this relationship a secret from everyone except her play therapist. She struggled to comprehend the polarities of staying involved with a person she felt finally understood her when she recognized that he was becoming increasingly callous and manipulative.

Several months after the beginning of their romantic involvement, Nichole ended her relationship with Cordell abruptly. Cordell was unhappy about this decision and sent Nichole an e-mail stating that he hoped she killed herself. He went on to say that when he killed himself, it would be her fault for breaking up with him. Nichole was distressed both for her own physical safety and for Cordell's well-being. Finally, school officials noticed the palpable changes in Nichole as her mood became depressed and irritable. It was during this critical time that Nichole also reported that her self-injurious behaviors had resumed and intensified in frequency. Nichole's parents reported noticing that she fluctuated between states of being irate and socially withdrawn but were confused by a set of separation anxiety symptoms that were emerging simultaneously. For example, Nichole refused to let her mother go away to visit family out of town. But once her mother agreed to stay home, Nichole vacillated between loving and hate-filled behaviors episodically, which is consistent with the *insecure ambivalent/resistant* attachment type. She yelled at her mother and refused to speak with her civilly for the entire weekend, castigating her at every chance that arose.

Jungian Play Therapy Approaches to Promote Secure Attachment

Although attachment relationships are thought to be relatively stable over time (Allan, 1988), they are indeed revisable within the context of new relationships. For many adolescents who enter play therapy, their experiences of empathy have been limited or disrupted in their early relationships (Green, Crenshaw & Langtiw, 2009). Thus, play therapy affords adolescents an opportunity to experience a secure, close relationship with a caring individual in which empathy, nonjudgmentalism, and permissiveness are hallmarks of the therapeutic alliance. Indeed, research has found that the value of the therapeutic relationship is greater than the value of specific interventions utilized in play therapy for youth and improves the quality of future relationships (Green, Crenshaw & Langtiw, 2009).

It is critically important that play therapists demonstrate their dependability early in treatment, through *empathic attunement* (listening carefully and empathizing accurately within the adolescents' phenomenological perspective) and *containment of distress* with clear boundaries (Reyes et al., 2010). Nichole shared with her therapist that some of the most memorable and successful sessions were those in the first few months, during which the play therapist simply sat with her while she expressed difficult emotions through her artwork and sandplay scenes. She told the play therapist that, over time, she felt less ashamed of her feelings and less afraid that the play therapist would think she was "weak" or "crazy." This view of a secure *Self*, which manifested itself in her relationships with peers, parents, and siblings, is largely what caused her self-injurious behaviors to desist. It was after she developed trust within the therapeutic relationship that she was able to begin containing her own emotions. During one particularly powerful session, Nichole engaged in an imagery-based containment exercise in which she visualized a safe and secure place where a container with a lock was located. The play therapist utilized guided imagery, accompanied by relaxation music, followed by an artistic exercise in which Nichole would creatively and abstractly paint the emotions felt throughout the imagery exercise. Following this session, Nichole regularly referred to her container and the way she felt safe to open it during her play therapy sessions.

From the beginning of the relationship, play therapists offer insecurely attached clients an opportunity to openly work through difficult feelings of disillusionment and abandonment through the consistency and dependability of the therapist and the therapeutic framework. That is, play therapists demonstrate unconditional congruence, empathy, and predictability in their words and actions. Further, it is the play therapist's responsibility to regularly explore and resolve anxieties within the transference and the client's experience of it. An example of this occurred with Nichole when her play therapist vacationed at the time period that paralleled her high school's final exams. Nichole expressed her resentment about feeling abandoned by the play therapist and her worries that the play therapist might not return from the vacation. Nichole created a sand world where she enacted a symbolic scene with magic stones and fairy princesses similar to what was occurring in her psyche regarding feeling let down that her therapist was vacationing during her finals. In this case, sandplay was beneficial because it permitted Nichole to express her frustration and freed her from anxieties so that she could generate viable alternatives on her own. The therapist did no verbal processing of the sand world after it was completed, but he honored the work through silence and acceptance.

Similarly, while Ilene struggled with the idea of going to a distant college where she might not be able to continue therapy, she found that journaling between sessions not only allowed her to feel a continued connectedness to her play therapist but also enabled her to openly reflect on her conflicting feelings. Writing these feelings down on paper was less threatening than directly talking about them. During one session, she spent much of the session drawing a series of self-portraits to make her journal a picture journal that represented her sense of self when alone, with her family members, and with the therapist.

In addition to these play-based activities, many creative adolescents spontaneously wish to write stories or letters to important figures in their lives (Green, 2012a). In these cases, the attempt to demonstrate feelings of attachment through play therapy interventions may be viewed as progress in the area of developing and sharing newfound ideas on nurturing attachment. Play therapists may choose to *process* (or discuss in depth) this with their clients, as many adolescents may feel thwarted to share the contents directly with the person involved. This feature promotes the expression of warm feelings engendered in emotionally safe relationships and encourages the building of healthy attachments (Crenshaw, 2008). The following section of the chapter describes a guided imagery activity that promotes the expression of contained symbols and emotions.

A Jungian Activity with Adolescents: My Guardian Spirit

A central archetypal drive during the adolescent phase of development is that of separation from the family of origin and the related sense of attachment. One function of separation is to attain one's own unique identity. The Guardian Spirit guided imagery technique has been modified from

Allan and Bertoia (1992). This guided imagery involves symbols inherent in such psychological functions as separating from the family of origin, purification of the body, overcoming childhood fears, death of the "old" childhood identity, learning new coping skills, and the birth of new inner and outer identities (Allan & Bertoia, 1992). Guided imagery activities are particularly relevant to adolescents because they provide a nonthreatening mechanism of entering the great search for and integration of the inscape of one's pure emotions. Jung (1964) termed this *individuation*.

The adolescent is prepared for the guided imagery activity through a few moments in relaxation techniques. Then the therapist reads:

> Close your eyes and let your mind wander for a while. . . . Now imagine that you are living many, many years ago . . . long before White people came to this land . . . and it is approaching time for you to leave on your Vision Quest in search of your Guardian Spirit. Let's get you a home base first: Where are you living? Who is in your family? . . . What does your lodge look like? . . . Now imagine a dream, and in the dream you become aware that it is time for you to leave your lodge and make your solo journey away from your home to find your Guardian Spirit. . . . Imagine leaving and walking for a long, long time . . . away from your home into the unknown countryside. . . . What do you see? . . . What is the weather like? After walking for a long time, you become aware that you are ready to begin your Vision Quest. To do this, you must find a safe and protected space. Soon you begin dreaming or imagining. . . . You're seeking a vision of your Guardian Spirit. Who comes to you? What is he, she, or it like? Continue dreaming for a while. . . . Picture the animal, person, or thing closely. Notice the details. . . . What noise does it make? What size and shape is it? What color is it? Picture yourself and your Guardian Spirit. What is it doing? What actions or words does it have for you? See if it leads you anywhere or shows or gives you anything. . . . Do you have any questions of it? . . . Let yourself ask. . . . Let him or her answer. . . . Now it is time to say goodbye to your Guardian Spirit. When you are ready lift your head and slowly open your eyes. . . . Now I'd like you to draw your Guardian Spirit and a scene from your inner journey and then we'll discuss.

This activity may open the adolescent's mind up to uniquely emotional experiences related to the process of identity formation (Allan & Bertoia, 1992). These inner experiences, when accompanied by drawings, may be highly influential in the lives of adolescents and facilitate the connection to depth, symbols, and the alchemical gold, or emotional richness, that waits within.

Clinical Implications for Jungian Play Therapists

One way play therapists can effectively begin therapy is to verify the attachment issues underlying the adolescents' problematic behaviors or their ineffective views of relationships with others. Being able to directly observe adolescents' attachment relationships with parents in sessions as well as to inquire about parents' and adolescents' views of trust, security, and communication in their current relationship may give the play therapist an impression of the quality of the attachment from both perspectives. In this way, parents are seen as *consultants* in the treatment process.

Witnessing the way in which parents and adolescents communicate information to the play therapist is often clinically significant. Noticing dynamics of the relationship, including who executes most of the verbalizations and how differences in opinions are communicated, for example, may be clinically beneficial. In secure relationships, teenagers are able to freely express their thoughts, feelings, and views of the presenting issues without anxiety that parents will reject them or withdraw nurturing (Reyes et al., 2010). However, in an insecure relationship, adolescents may struggle with anxiety or low self-esteem, failing to view their contributions as worthwhile and frequently looking to their parents to lead them toward the correct answers (Black et al., 2010; McGee et al., 2006). Finally, understanding the role that others play in adolescents' lives is inherently important when determining the most effective treatment plan and play-based interventions to incorporate. Insecure attachment can manifest itself in a number of ways, ranging from an overreliance in relationships or unhealthy development of friendships and romantic partners, to a "loner" stance, where attachment relationships are minimized and reliance on others avoided. If the information gathered from the parent-teen dyad suggests an unhealthy attachment that is affecting the adolescent's internal or external world, the play therapist may choose to work directly with this dynamic through family play therapy and possibly family sandplay (Green & Connolly, 2009).

Another key implication in Jungian Play Therapy with adolescents to strengthen attachment is that a healthy play therapist–adolescent client relationship is characterized by mutual trust and respect (Eliot, 2009). Research on therapeutic relationships suggests that the emotional bond between an adolescent and a play therapist is the key to lasting and productive change within the psychotherapy (Black et al., 2010). By framing the play therapy session with specific limits and boundaries, therapists assist adolescents in learning that the dyad is psychologically safe. Specifically, adolescents internalize safety and security as they are able to express and direct raw, honest emotions directly or symbolically without being judged or asked to change parts of themselves that others may see as unacceptable or undesirable. The unconditional acceptance gleaned from such an experience may be different from what adolescents experience in their peer or parental relationships (Castro-Blanco & Karver, 2010).

It can make a significant difference in the frequency and openness of emotional expressiveness for perfectionistic teens to be permitted to act playfully or aggressively within the safety of a nonjudgmental attachment between themselves and a play therapist. Play therapists may also wish to incorporate the research supporting the view that therapy gains made early on are based upon the contribution of a strong alliance (McGee et al., 2006; Reyes et al., 2010). Forming a caring therapeutic dyad early on in adolescent treatment may be challenging for play therapists who are also trying to formulate a positive, working relationship with the parents (who may be despised by the adolescent). It seems that the primary responsibility is for the therapist to focus on building a relationship with the adolescent before working with the family (Berlin & Cassidy, 1999).

Another key implication for play therapists regarding attachment is that some adolescents strive to cultivate a rich interior life in relation to their most significant relationships, including the play therapist. Adolescents' positive psychological growth is contingent upon intimate, secure, safe relationships in which they can express their individuality without judgment; many at-risk adolescents lack such relationships (Perl, 2008). Sandplay and other expressive art therapy interventions may be conduits for adolescents to express themselves and their world to the play therapist in less threatening ways. Through these sand pictures and other creative expressions, adolescents come to understand (a) that their feelings are of value, (b) that they are supported by caring adults who do not judge them, and (c) that attention to their inner emotional landscape is a vital key to their ongoing psychological development.

Through the unique unconditional acceptance in the Jungian Play Therapy relationship, some adolescents come to realize that they may thrive with the support of caring adults to help them overcome obstacles, solve problems, take responsibility, and make meaningful contributions to their schools and home communities. However, many adolescents who come into the consulting room are in families and communities that expect little of them in terms of social interest. Many are not mentored by caring, competent adults, and they seem to possess an incongruent sense of personal responsibility to their family, neighbors, and social networks (Green, Schweiker, et al., 2009). These disaffected adolescents are often unsure of their place in the world and do not believe in their value to society. Children and adolescents respond positively to play therapists who actively and nonjudgmentally listen to them and provide supportive and creative ways to help them understand themselves, including play therapy interventions like sandplay that may promote secure attachment (Donald, 2003; Green & Connolly, 2009; Kestley, 2010).

Through the unique unconditional acceptance in the play therapy relationship, some adolescents may come to a *corrective emotional experience* (Black et al., 2010), particularly when adolescents' real life experiences have been contaminated by tragic loss, trauma, broken and inconsistent relationships, and a lack of stable attachments. Although there are no specific research-based play interventions to immediately and/or comprehensively resolve the effects of broken attachment, the most current attachment research demonstrates that a relationship with a securely attached significant adult can enable an adolescent to become more securely attached and view her world, once again, as more stable, secure, and safe (Castro-Blanco & Karver, 2010; Crenshaw, 2008; Green, 2012a; McGee et al., 2006).

III JUNGIAN PLAY THERAPY

Applications

6

With Children Affected by Sexual Abuse

The dark night of the soul comes just before revelation. When everything is lost, and all seems dark, then comes the new life, and all that is needed.

—Joseph Campbell

_____

Child sexual abuse (CSA) is a pervasive, traumatic event (Heflin & Deblinger, 2007) affecting hundreds of thousands of ethnically and socioeconomically diverse children and families across the United States (Putnam, 2003). Gil (2006) and Shelby and Felix (2005) have noted that integrative therapies—those that combine directive and nondirective strategies—possess the capacity to benefit a child traumatized by sexual assault. Jungian Play Therapy (JPT) is one such integrative therapy that may be beneficial when applied to children affected by CSA. Within the safety of a nonjudgmental, therapeutic relationship, children affected by CSA may become consciously aware of and subsequently resolve conflicting emotions associated with sexual assault in symbolic, less-threatening ways. This chapter presents a case study of a sexually abused child, showing how the Jungian play process, as well as the relationship, paved the way for a meaningful trauma integration to occur.

In the United States, there have been several nationally publicized accounts recently of child sex abuse involving (a) teachers' sexual misconduct with children in American public schools (Maxwell & Holovach, 2007), (b) an isolated cross-section of ministers and clergy fondling and/or raping young children while working for churches and faith-based organizations (De-Cosse, 2007; Dunne, 2004), and (c) online predators luring children into las-civious acts behind the veil of anonymity afforded by the Internet (Marcum, 2007). After decades of denial, shame, and compartmentalization (Deb-linger & Runyon, 2005), Western culture has begun to notice and react to the alarming prevalence of CSA by invoking tougher laws against sexual pred-ators (Gaines, 2006; Levenson et al., 2007) and by removing some of the social stigmatization associated with the survivors of CSA (Schultz, 2005). One unfortunate outcome of more strident judicial policies against child molesters in the United States is that some pedophiles are now migrating to countries where they can purchase sex from minors with little or no polic-ing by local authorities (Barnitz, 2001). These recent developments in the perpetuation of CSA highlight the importance of play therapists becoming conversant and competent in current trauma-focused interventions when counseling this special population.

Hetzel-Riggin, Brausch, and Montgomery (2007) evaluated 28 studies in a meta-analysis that provided treatment outcome results for sexually abused children and adolescents. Different aspects of psychological treatment, such as specific treatment modalities (e.g., play therapy or cognitive behavioral therapy), were investigated. The results indicated that psychological treat-ment after CSA resulted in better outcomes than no treatment. Play therapy was the most effective treatment for improving children's social function-ing, whereas cognitive behavioral, abuse-specific, and supportive therapy in either group or individual format was most effective in ameliorating problematic externalizing behaviors. These results illuminate the need for a treatment modality to emphasize creativity and the therapeutic relation-ship, which are typically involved in play therapy and expressive therapies (i.e., sand therapy and art therapy), as well as directive techniques associ-ated with shaping behaviors and correcting children's misattributions.

Jungian Play Therapy (JPT) is a creative, play-based treatment approach that both meets traumatized children where they are developmentally and integrates more directive techniques to help reshape disordered behaviors. This chapter (a) provides a brief overview of the prevalence and conse-quences of CSA; (b) outlines the central tenets of a Jungian play approach to counseling children traumatized by sexual violence; (c) includes a case study to illustrate JPT's application with CSA; and (d) provides a post-analysis and conclusion.

Prevalence and Psychological Sequelae

CSA is a pervasive trend of victimization in the United States, often resulting in protracted, adverse psychological effects (Briere & Elliot, 2003; Briere & Scott, 2006; Gil, 2006). Recent epidemiological studies have depicted the CSA incidence rates over the past several years as averaging 27% for adult women and 16% for adult men (U.S. Department of Health & Human Services, 2006). However, the actual number of cases is disputable because the figures underestimate the actual rates of CSA. One reason for the various disparities in number of CSA reports is that the legal definition of CSA varies between states, thereby creating many operational definitions that influence prevalence statistics. Also, many cases go unreported and therefore are unknown to professionals. For clarity, in this chapter, I adopted Cohen, Mannarino, and Deblinger's (2006) definition of CSA as sexual exploitation involving physical contact between a child and another person in which (a) exploitation implies an inequality of power between the child and the abuser and (b) physical contact includes anal, genital, oral, or breast contact.

According to Briere and Scott (2006), sexually abused children may experience a variety of traumatic stressors, including the constellation of symptoms associated with Post-Traumatic Stress Disorder (PTSD). Some of these stressors may include intrusive memories or re-experiencing the traumatic event, as witnessed in children through repetitive themes of reenactment of the trauma in play behaviors, hyper-arousal, and avoidance of stimuli associated with the trauma (Hunter, 2006; Widom, 1999). For example, a retrospective study of elementary-school-age boys indicated that sexually abused boys presented more persistently over time with a variety of ailments akin to PTSD, including frightening nightmares, than their nonabused peers (Maddocks et al., 1999). Although there is no evidence in the literature of a clear post–sexual abuse syndrome, studies have shown that 50% of children affected by CSA exhibit symptoms of PTSD and 32% to 48% meet full criteria for a PTSD diagnosis (Heflin & Deblinger, 2007). Another study has shown that 40% of children affected by CSA demonstrated measurable symptoms (Finkelhor & Berliner, 1995). Typically, researchers have found that sexually abused children are affected adversely emotionally, behaviorally, and academically in both the short and the long term (Rowe & Eckenrode, 1999; Webster, 2001; Widom, 1999). Additionally, cognitive misattributions, feelings of terror and helplessness, stigmatization, and abuse-specific internal attributions resulting from CSA have been associated with elevated levels of distress and psychopathology in children (Heflin & Deblinger, 2007).

CSA appears to be linked to cycles of violence in minors as some sexually abused children abuse other minors (Marshall, 1997). Moreover, some sexually abused children go on to be abused as adults (Gil, 2006). Although it is important to note that a subsection of CSA victims does not show immediate or apparent psychological or behavioral difficulties, this perceived lack of symptoms could be related to denial or shock (Webster, 2001). There is support for the idea that denial or shock causes sleeper effects; research has shown that as time passes, some survivors of CSA begin to demonstrate psychological and behavioral disturbances in adulthood (Widom, 1999).

Treatment Approaches

The gold standard of trauma-focused interventions, or the treatment modality that empirically demonstrates a reduction in disordered behaviors associated with PTSD and other trauma-specific variables and behaviors affiliated with CSA, is cognitive behavioral therapy (CBT) and trauma-focused CBT (Cohen et al., 2006; Deblinger et al., 2006; Heflin & Deblinger, 2007). These evidence-based approaches combine children's retelling or reliving aspects of the abuse (e.g., gradual exposure and affective processing) with nonoffending parental psycho-education (e.g., behavior management skills). One limitation of CBT is its reliance on a child's ability to (a) use cognitive and verbal functioning skills, (b) use acute reasoning, (c) identify motivations to alter behaviors, and (d) engage in accountability. Children may be incapable developmentally or emotionally of participating successfully in verbal-based interventions. Furthermore, "a desired change in a child's behavior may be achieved, but this may occur in isolation from . . . understanding or true processing" (Gil, 2006, p. 101). From a Jungian perspective, CBT and trauma-focused CBT are standardized, clinical approaches that may be uncomfortable for children who use denial as a defensive mechanism to protect their fragile ego against the assaults from sexual trauma, especially those affronted by CSA. These children may not have the "ego-strength" to cognitively resolve traumatic events. Two evidence-informed play therapy models, trauma-focused play therapy (Gil, 2006) and post-traumatic play therapy (Shelby & Felix, 2005), use a prescriptive, modularized approach with child sexual assault survivors that includes active learning principles and experiential activities with caretakers (Shelby, 2007). Gil (2006), Shelby and Felix (2005), and Rasmussen and Cunningham (1995) wrote about the effectiveness of an integrative treatment with abused and traumatized children—combining trauma-focused, empirical-based directive models and nondirective or expressive play therapies. Expressive therapies, such as JPT, combine gradual exposure and affective work within the safety of an engaged, nonjudgmental, therapeutic relationship.

JPT is one hybrid of creative and integrative therapies: it follows some of the tenets espoused through the child-centered, nondirective protocol: (a) children know where they need to go emotionally to heal themselves and (b) building a trusting, nonevaluative therapeutic relationship is essential. JPT differs from pure nondirective therapy in that it permits a therapist the freedom to incorporate directive activities (Allan, 1988; Green, 2007) to isolate specific disordered behaviors associated with abuse and resolve inherent difficulties associated with reactive symptoms. Three Jungian interventions demonstrated to reduce anxiety associated with certain features of traumatic experiences include (a) the coloring of mandalas (Henderson et al., 2007), (b) creating a trauma narrative via sandplay (Allan, 1988), and (c) utilizing fairy tales with guided imagery to decrease hyper-arousal (Green & Ironside, 2004). JPT provides an analytical attitude and depth of understanding of symbols and their meaning, which may ultimately benefit a child assimilating post-trauma.

Jungian Play Techniques with CSA

One of the basic premises of JPT is that children express their perceptions of the world most easily through graphic representations, such as picture drawings or symbolic play under metaphorical guises (Allan, 1988; Landreth, 2002; Oaklander, 1978). According to Piaget (1962), the symbolic function of play with children bridges the gap between concrete experience and abstract thought most efficiently. Children understand the world through visual and symbolic methods. Through play therapy, children may regulate their inner world by projecting difficult feelings and images onto objects in an emotionally safe and protected space. Jungian play therapists use different symbolic interventions, such as serial drawings, spontaneous drawings, and picture journals to engage the child in expressing wishes and repressed emotions.

Serial drawings refer to a child's drawing weekly in the presence of a therapist, with the therapist analyzing the drawings as a monolithic series over time (Allan & Bertoia, 1992). A sequence of drawings encourages the expression of the child's self-healing archetype through symbolic language depiction, which may facilitate inner conflict resolution. Serial drawings are the avenue to amplifying symbols that appear in children's artwork, especially self-healing symbols that are necessary to activate adaptive coping responses. For example, a sexually abused 11-year-old child named Joe exhibited intrusive re-experiencing of his biological mother's sexually assaulting him when he was 10 years old. He slept intermittently, often waking in the night from bad dreams, with no recognizable content in the dream to discern. The play therapist instructed Joe to draw a tree; he drew a hole in the middle of the tree and colored it black. After Joe completed the drawing, the therapist asked, "Joe, if you were inside there [the therapist pointed to the hole in the tree but did not label it], what might you be feeling?" Joe responded, "Happy, because I would be with the owl that lives in the tree." The therapist restated, "So you would be content because you were in a safe place with a friend you like." Then Joe replied, "Yes, and I would have a flashlight so the tree goblins wouldn't hurt us." After several more sessions of serial drawings, the therapist guided Joe to draw images of light illuminating darkness (amplification of symbols). Joe's legal caretakers commented to the therapist how Joe began sleeping with a night light on in his room, and his nightmares attenuated.

Picture journaling is used when counseling elementary-school-age children affected by sexual assault because it permits children to reflect on their developmental processes by combining journal writing and artistic creations (Allan & Brown, 1993). In this technique children maintain a picture journal between sessions. Children produce the journal via artistic creations using colored pencils. The therapist instructs children to create pictures regarding important events or feelings in their journal and asks them to bring the journal to the play therapy sessions. From a Jungian perspective, picture journaling assists children in extracting meaning from their assault by reconnecting to or discovering a rich interior life. Once the self-healing archetype surfaces, children will identify the archetype and the feelings associated with the archetype as they permeate throughout the emotional landscape. This process was seen in the sun/light image with Joe. The image tells children where they need to go emotionally for healing, and the therapist trusts that a *vis naturalis* (a natural life force) is working via the *participation mystique* (the connection between the child's mind and body) to help release the power and emotion of living in an unconscious, mythical underworld. Picture journaling combines the therapeutic activity of creating a trauma narrative with symbolic pictures, which may release children's emotional blocks to repressed traumatic material.

Spontaneous drawing is a semi-directive technique that helps children affected by CSA to express their thoughts and feelings in nonthreatening or less-threatening mechanisms (Allan, 1988; Green & Hebert, 2006). The purpose of spontaneous drawing is to provide children an emotionally and physically safe therapeutic environment in which they exhibit self-control and mastery by choosing their own ideas for drawing. With autonomy, clients are allowed to symbolically and artistically abreact repressed emotional anguish stemming from their trauma-specific event (Kalsched, 1996). As critical issues appear during the course of treatment—psychological reactivity, emotional numbing, and dissociation—the therapist may choose a more directive technique. The therapist may choose a grounding activity germane to the client's psychosocial healing and adaptation to the traumatic event. When using spontaneous drawings in play therapy, the therapist says to the client, "Please draw whatever you'd like." The client chooses the content to draw; perceptual distortions, reenactment of the trauma, and regressions may appear in the child's artwork (Allan, 1988; Allan & Bertoia, 1992; Furth, 1988; Green & Hebert, 2006). Moreover, symbols from the unconscious appear in spontaneous drawings, expressing the psyche's need for healing through fantasy. These symbols, called *compensatory symbols,* illustrated through spontaneous drawings, may ultimately foster healing through psychic integration and balance. Compensatory symbols may bridge the neglected areas of the unconscious to conscious awareness. Identification with salubrious symbols in play therapy activates the healing potential that exists within the child; thus, the self-healing archetype emerges.

The Self-Healing Archetype

A Jungian play therapist facilitates the traumatized child's activation of the self-healing archetype by encouraging creativity and energy associated with the unconscious symbol. Specifically, the symbol tells children where they are by pointing to the area of the unconscious that is most neglected, and the therapist unconditionally accepts that position. After the self-healing symbol appears in play, the therapist explores the child's inner language by reconciling the meaning of the symbol using a phenomenological perspective. Play therapists assist traumatized children in reconciling the meaning of the symbol by (a) asking what the symbol means and (b) externalizing the accompanying inner dialogue associated with the symbol.

Typically, this is more effective with children older than age 8 because of developmental and cognitive considerations. For example, if a 9-year-old child draws variations of a rainbow, the therapist may first ask the child what the rainbow means. Second, the therapist may attempt to amplify (explore) the symbol by asking the child questions or making comments such as, "Let's talk about each of the colors and what they mean to the rainbow. Which color does the rainbow like best/least?" "Where was the rainbow before the scene occurred?" or "What makes the rainbow come out and shine with these bright colors?" With the emptying of all preconceived notions of the meaning of symbols, play therapists facilitate an open path for children to experience their own inner healing. If a child is younger than 8, the reconciliation of the meaning of the symbol may perhaps be inferred through drawing analysis and viewing the gestalt of the child's psychology.

Case Illustration

An 18-year-old male relative sexually assaulted Lily, an 8-year-old Native American girl living in a subsided housing section of an urban city in the southern United States. Lily was molested on weekends over six months while her mother was working. The perpetrator assaulted Lily repeatedly and asked her to keep it a secret. He emotionally and verbally manipulated her through fear by stating that the police would be called and remove Lily from her mother's home if anyone found out about the sexual assaults. This paralyzed Lily with fear, because she and her mother lived alone and their extended family was located in another part of the country. Lily was dependent on her mother for all of her financial, emotional, and practical needs. Lily's father died when she was 3 years old from a gunshot wound related to gang activity, and her mother worked two part-time jobs to maintain their household.

While the abuse occurred, Lily's grades declined and her behaviors at home and with female peers became disordered. She displayed avoidance of trauma-related stimuli by becoming hyper-aroused around adult men. Specifically, she became defiant when attending science class, taught by Mr. Smith, the only male teacher at Lily's elementary school. Eventually, Lily disclosed the sexual abuse to a female teacher, and a child protective agency was notified. After the forensic interview, child protective services referred

Lily to a play therapist. On intake, her presenting problems were (a) numbing of her general responsiveness at school and at home and (b) defiant behaviors in Mr. Smith's class.

Lily's therapist used spontaneous drawings from the initial counseling session to develop the therapeutic relationship and begin the extended developmental assessment (EDA), which lasted approximately 11 sessions. The EDA (Gil, 2006) is a comprehensive and sensitive assessment that involves (a) a caretaker intake with a complete cognitive behavioral assessment of the child; (b) obtaining historical, medical, and behavioral traits of the child post- and pre-abuse; and (c) conducting 8–12 individual play sessions, using both directive and nondirective assessments and play-based methods to inform and initiate treatment planning. Throughout the EDA, the therapist observed Lily's artistic abilities. Lily symbolically depicted many of the issues related to CSA that she had difficulty expressing orally. For example, Lily drew images of a white, magnificent castle surrounded by a moat that was excavated for additional fortification. Her drawings typically contained a bright yellow sun, and smiling, beautiful fairy princesses appeared in the castle's windows. Staying with the metaphor, the play therapist asked Lily what the fairy princesses were viewing outside the window. Lily replied, "They are waiting for a handsome prince to come and marry them. He will be nice to them, and they will be happy."

The play therapist observed that Lily's drawings and verbalizations of the meanings of the drawings conveyed *wish fulfillment*, which possibly depicted her need to feel love in a safe, nonsexualized way. Lily inserted a dark, unicorn-like figure looming behind one or more trees in many of her drawings. Moreover, Lily reported that the dark figure was "an evil unicorn trying to hurt people with his horn because he was hungry and wanted food." The therapist further amplified the symbol of the dark unicorn by asking Lily to draw a new picture with the same castle but with a unicorn that had enough food and did not need to puncture anyone with his horn. She drew a unicorn that found berries and nuts on the ground, and his color changed from dark and ominous to a lighter, more whimsical brown. She then appeared less intense; her affect changed from serious and concerned to relieved as she began to regain mastery and control of her feelings. Without a probe from the therapist, Lily replied, "My uncle was bad and used to hurt me, and I used to be scared. I always thought it was my fault because he told me it was. But now he's hurting 'cause he's in trouble for what he did to me, and it was bad. But I'm not bad." After talking about the pictures and exploring her individual perspective, the play therapist conceptualized Lily's drawings as internalizing positive effects of hope and stability in a fantastic, mythical world that she created. She also began to articulate her trauma narrative and no longer self-victimized or self-blamed.

This example demonstrated the notion of *intrinsic processing* through reexperiencing the traumatic event (Briere & Scott, 2006). Specifically, Lily's mind repeatedly relived disturbing features or memories of the trauma symbolically through her drawings, which may have represented an evolutionally derived attempt to promote cognitive and affective accommodation to the reality of the trauma. By systematically desensitizing or extinguishing emotions and cognitions from the event through mastery of the feelings and thoughts associated with it, Lily's conditioned responses to the traumatic event changed. This clinical opinion follows the trauma theory promulgated by Briere and Scott (2006) that stipulates that emotional processing of traumatic events occurs when "erroneous perceptions, beliefs, and expectations ('pathological fear structures') associated with trauma-related fears are activated and habituated in the context of new, more accurate information" (p. 121). In other words, because Lily resolved painful emotional material in the presence of a nonjudgmental therapist and was able to pair positive emotions and cognitions with painful, previous trauma-relevant stimuli, she experienced meaningful trauma integration.

JPT Goals: Treating Sexual Trauma in Children

One of the primary goals of JPT is to restore a child to pre-abuse functioning. The spontaneous drawing technique was a significant component of Lily's EDA because it informed the treatment planning. Lily seemed to begin the process of restoring hope to her insecure outlook on life through individual creative expression in the presence of a caring counselor. Lily conveyed her unconscious or tacit psychic longings to be loved in a safe way through spontaneous drawings in a nonjudgmental, therapeutic relationship. In several of her drawings, she illustrated and seemed connected to one or more of the fairy princesses, and her self-healing archetype emerged.

After sitting with, or contemplating, the images and providing the therapist with her own interpretation of the images in the drawings, Lily began to internalize feelings of security and contentment. Previously, these feelings were compromised by the sexual assault. Once Lily internalized positive cognitive attributions of her world as stable, meaningful, and ordered and connected those internalizations to her outer world, Lily's reactive symptoms began to dissipate. Combined with several cognitive behavioral strategies such as cognitive restructuring and disputing irrational beliefs about Lily's complicity in the abuse, Lily and her therapist made slow progress in reducing Lily's emotional numbing and cognitive distortions. Lily's mother and teacher, through filial therapy and consultation, respectively, began praising Lily for her prosocial behaviors and offering suggestions for coping mechanisms when she became distraught. The teacher expressed concern to the therapist that because the school did not perform any type of psycho-education to children regarding fending off sexual predators or normalizing the disclosure process, this may have contributed to Lily's abuse continuing for several months. The teacher, collaborating with the therapist, petitioned for a new psycho-educational program on CSA to the school's principal and the county, and both were approved for execution. Also, Lily's teacher and school counselor conveyed that their skills were augmented after their consultations with the therapist. They brokered peer relationships by conducting more group work in class and placing Lily with young girls who were psychologically adjusted and socially appropriate. Lily developed the capacity to reach out to her same-sex peers and re-form friendships, and she began evidencing an elevation in pro-social behaviors and an increased level of positive peer interaction.

A second goal of JPT with children affected by CSA is to facilitate resilience through the recognition and utilization of effective coping mechanisms. The traditional paradigm of counseling children that uses talking methods, often associated with adult psychotherapy, is often insufficient to guide abused children through self-healing (Gil, 2006; Green & Christensen, 2006; Landreth et al., 1999). Spontaneous drawings are a nonverbal technique used in JPT because drawings assist children in artistically externalizing emotions stemming from sexual assault. Drawings and interpretations of drawings may enable the child's psyche to consciously identify the self-healing potential that talking alone cannot accomplish. Through spontaneous drawings and the contemplation of symbols, Lily identified with the beautiful and happy fairy princesses who were safe in the castle and protected behind a moat. These princesses and the prince may have represented Lily reconciling the anima and animus archetypes (female traits within a male, and male traits within a female, respectively) that had been activated by the premature sexual encounter. Her identification of the self-healing archetype encouraged coping mechanisms, such as her ability to be light-hearted with a sense of humor to handle pain, something that had lain dormant since the assault.

The third central goal of JPT is to incorporate nonoffending caretakers in family play therapy and to coordinate services with other significant adults in the child's home, school, and community through consultation and collaboration. Lily's therapist evaluated her environmental support structures, and a multi-disciplinary team was formed to assist Lily and her family following the crisis of the CSA disclosure. The therapist met with (a) Lily's academic teachers, including Mr. Smith; (b) ancillary support staff, including her resource specialist; (c) medical and mental health personnel (e.g., the school nurse and the social worker); and (d) administrative staff (e.g., the assistant principal) to answer the questions they posed on the potential behavioral effects of CSA. The school team also cooperated on formulating practical solutions to complex issues, such as allowing Lily to switch science classes until she felt comfortable returning to a classroom with a male teacher, which she eventually did. Also, Lily's mother attended family therapy sessions with the play therapist and the child every three weeks. During these sessions, the play therapist listened to the mother's concerns, validated her feelings, and provided practical strategies to increase her patience with and understanding of the healing process. In addition, the mother and the child drew together, sanded pictures, and played.

Analysis and Conclusion

Throughout the clinical process of bridging the unconscious to the conscious, Lily's self-healing archetype became activated by the therapeutic relationship. Lily's self-healing archetype emerged when she shared her drawings in the presence of an accepting, permissive therapist. After six months of weekly individual psychotherapy sessions, Lily's therapist, teachers, and family noticed a decrease in her emotional pain and a reduction in her morbid self-alienation stemming from the shame she felt regarding the sexual assault.

At the beginning of treatment, Lily began to self-heal her emotional wounds while smoothing out the roughness of her exterior—evidenced by her improvement in grades and increased social connections. Part of this process involved Lily's ability to reconcile her dysphoric outer world with her turbulent inner world. This occurred partially because the play therapist articulated to Lily that the abuse was just one small part of who she was and did not define who she was. Lily eventually internalized this accurate appraisal. Lily created several picture journals of all of the pieces that made her who she was, not just the assault, and this began to change her self-concept positively. After the defensive splitting lost its negative valence in Lily's psyche, the negative effects associated with the trauma appeared, and she began to resolve the internalized guilt. The guilt, stemming from her cognitive misattributions of culpability in the sexual assault, manifested externally as emotional numbing and defiance in a male teacher's classroom setting.

Once the recognition of opposites occurred within the protection of the therapeutic relationship, Lily felt empowered and engaged in positive self-talk, "This [therapy] wasn't so bad after all, and I feel better now and know that what he did to me was not my fault." Furthermore, the therapeutic relationship facilitated Lily's inner healing because of the frequency of the play therapist's affirmations—consistent verbal acknowledgments of Lily's heroic struggle to overcome self-condemnation. The play therapist's affirmations were praises of Lily's efforts: "Lily, you are placing so much effort and energy into this exercise. I just wanted to acknowledge that I appreciate your commitment to this process, even though I know it may be scary at times. I can't say for sure I know how things will work out, and I don't know if everything will be OK. But I do know that I will be here with you."

Lily became aware of the slow, numinous transformation going on within. From a Jungian point of view, Lily had relied on the transcendent power of the Self to counter-condition pain and desolation invoked by the sexual assault, to formulate accurate cognitive appraisals and symbolic interpretations of the event. The new feelings and healthy images associated with the event allowed Lily to generate a new perspective. In an archetypal underworld, Lily felt free to integrate conflicting symbols and images associated with the assault to produce a more accurate, meaningful trauma narrative.

From a Jungian viewpoint, Lily found solace within a therapeutic relationship, where pain and fear transformed to comfort and courage. As the Greek goddess Athena guided Telemachus to find his father, Odysseus, through a perilous journey, the play therapist accompanies the child into her underworld, to go *into the wounding*. To Jung, a relationship to the symbolic life is a prerequisite for growth and healing. Specifically, play therapists facilitate children's understanding of how they can relate to the symbols inside them. Post-traumatic growth occurs when children work with symbols within, as the Self leads the child to the healing, where safety, security, and stability await.

7

With Adolescents Who Have ADHD

How can I be substantial if I do not cast a shadow? I must have a
dark side also, if I am to be whole.

—Carl Jung

———

Adolescent males diagnosed with Attention-Deficit / Hyperactivity
Disorder (ADHD) typically present with symptoms related to social
difficulties, low self-esteem, and externalizing behavior problems.
The unique developmental and diagnostic-specific characteristics of adolescent males with ADHD make a verbal approach to
abstractions often difficult. Jungian Play Therapy (JPT) provides
a creative, potentially beneficial alternative to traditional talk or
cognitive therapy to remediate concerns associated with the ADHD
diagnosis. The current literature maintains a paucity of creative, developmentally appropriate play (or activity) therapies that mediate
typical issues associated with this population. The JPT techniques
of drawing and coloring mandalas offer a therapeutic alternative
for exploration when counseling adolescents (Baggerly & Green,
2013; Green, Drewes & Kominski, 2013). This chapter features an
overview of the current mental health literature on working with
adolescents diagnosed with ADHD. It also presents a case study to
demonstrate how coloring of mandalas may be a beneficial intervention in Jungian Play Therapy with adolescents.

Attention-Deficit / Hyperactivity Disorder (ADHD) is one of the most commonly diagnosed childhood disorders today, with reported rates ranging

from 3% to 12% of the total population (Buschgens et al., 2008; Froehlich et al., 2007). It is more prevalent in males than females, particularly in the diagnosis of the hyperactive/impulsive type (APA, 2000). Bryan, Burnstein and Ergul (2004) have explored social and emotional ramifications associated with special needs students, such as students with ADHD. The deficits that are characteristic of ADHD (i.e., deficits in memory, emotions, and behaviors) can cause adolescent males to experience psychosocial as well as educational difficulties in a typical classroom (Graetz et al., 2006). Specifically, many adolescents with ADHD lack the social networks that their peers and non-ADHD siblings enjoy (Buschgen et al., 2008).

Some adolescents who experience social difficulties display internalizing symptoms, such as anxiety and depressed affect, while others externalize their distress through aggressive or violent behaviors (Buschgens et al., 2008; APA, 2000). These minors are at greater risk for multiple psychiatric disorders such as depression, clinically significant anxiety, externalizing behavior disorders, affect dysregulation, illicit substance abuse and dependence, and suicidal ideation (Bryan et al., 2004; Kavale et al., 2005).

The Mandala as a Treatment Approach

A mandala is any piece of artwork that is created within a bound shape, customarily a circle (Henderson et al., 2007). *Mandala* is a Sanskrit word meaning "sacred circle" (Fincher, 2000). The circular shape of a mandala connotes wholeness and integration (see fig. 7.1). Mandalas can be found in the sacred artwork of cultures throughout time, from cave drawings and rock carvings to sand paintings and stained-glass windows. A mandala, or magic circle, is used as a meditative tool in various religions, but most famously in Tibetan Buddhism. The mandala circle (with inner symbolic patterns) may promote psychological healing through the calmness arising from a peaceful state of mind when a mandala is created by an individual (Mahar et al., 2012).

The use of the mandala as a therapeutic tool was first introduced by Giordono Bruno in the sixteenth century, then later by Carl Jung (1973), who suggested that the act of drawing a mandala had a calming and healing effect on its creator while at the same time facilitating psychic integration and personal meaning in life. Jung explored the psychological meaning of mandalas, viewing them as symbolic of the inner process from which individuals grow toward fulfilling their potential for wholeness. He surmised that

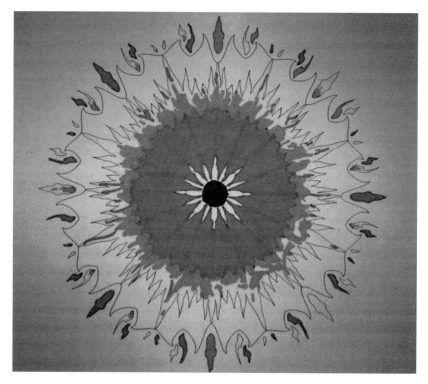

Figure 7.1. Mandala image in psychotherapy

the mandala was a manifestation of the individual psyche's self-regulating system, which helps to maintain orderly functioning and can, when needed, restore stability (Fincher, 2009). Jung saw in his clients' nonverbal creation of mandalas a natural process of generating and resolving inner conflicts that would bring about greater complexity, harmony, and stability in the personality.

The mandala functions as a symbolic representation of affective material constellated in the psyche yet unknown or unconscious to the individual; but at the same time the mandala provides a sense of order through concentration and integration to this material (Henderson, 2007). The power of such imaginative psychic concentration is used in modern psychotherapy; and its positive content is a therapeutic tool used in cognitive and behavioristic forms of psychotherapy as part of the relaxation principle. In situations of stress and fear, the concentrated visualization of a personal healing mandala can have protective effects on the individual, even helping to generate new patterns of protective processes and coping mechanisms (Bonny & Kellogg, 1977).

The main aspect of a meditative approach and activity, such as the use of the mandala with clients diagnosed with ADHD, is that it is a cognitive and intention-based process characterized by self-regulation and attention to the present moment with an open and accepting orientation toward one's experiences. This may result in improved attention and concentration as well as possibly offering symptom relief to adolescents coping with negative side effects associated with ADHD (Zylowska et al., 2008). By creating or coloring a mandala, the brain shifts more easily into a meditative state, an alpha wave frequency, which often results in an inner calmness and a relaxed state (Beaucaire, 2012). This meditative state occurs as the mandala is being created or colored or as it is observed. Consequently, the sense of inner peace, a potential correlation associated with the mandala's properties, may neutralize causes of stress and might help to reorder an adolescent's thoughts (Green & Drewes, 2013).

Jungian Play Therapy with ADHD Adolescent Males: The Research

Adolescence often comprises crises of identity with opportunities to experience growth toward individuation or "psychological wholeness" (Green, Drewes & Kominski, 2013; Patton, 2006). Jungian Play Therapy is a modality that presents adolescents with a symbolic, emotionally safe outlet to recover disowned or disconnected cognitions and emotions in less threatening ways than verbal interventions (Allan & Brown, 1993). This is particularly beneficial if the adolescent is unable to cognitively, verbally, or emotionally address difficult analytical material and would otherwise be overwhelmed by the associated emerging affect.

The use of the mandala, specifically, allows the adolescent with ADHD a nonverbal or less verbal approach with a healing, meditative effect. Adolescents can experience relaxation and psychological healing leading to a discovery of personal meaning through meditating on and/or creating mandalas (Henderson et al., 2007). In analytical terms, mandalas promote healing by facilitating intrapsychic communication between the *Self* and the *ego* through archetypal symbols and their associated or collective affective undertones. That which is unconscious is brought to consciousness through the creation of the mandala. Although there is little empirical research focusing on the use of mandalas as an effective mental health intervention specifically with ADHD adolescents, Henderson and colleagues' (2007) results provided initial empirical support that warrants further study. They found that a sample of individuals suffering from Post-Traumatic Stress Disorder experienced a reduction in trauma symptoms after they drew symbols and representations of their trauma and emotional response within mandalas. Henderson and colleagues note that case studies and clinical observations consistently support the efficacy of mandalas as a medium of healing, particularly in cases where the clients or patients are unable to express themselves verbally because of trauma, shame, or cognitive deficit.

Mandalas may be a beneficial tool for ADHD adolescents as they begin thinking about and expressing their thoughts and feelings in a safe and contained space. Mandalas were chosen by the therapist in the case study later in this chapter to use with the adolescent, over other types of expressive art therapy interventions, because the adolescent expressed an interest in the activity. The mandala sometimes helps the client to focus and center himself emotionally and cognitively into the task at hand, while allowing the therapeutic components of the experience to aid in emotional healing and integration (Fincher, 2009). The process of creating a mandala, as seen in this chapter's case example, helped the client to become more conscious of his inner thoughts and facilitated reflection and relaxation.

Coloring and/or creating mandalas has been used in mental health contexts with numerous populations and settings, including individuals with Post-Traumatic Stress Disorder and dissociative disorders (Cox & Cohen, 2000), traumatic grief (Henderson et al., 2007; Pizarro, 2004), and Attention-Deficit/Hyperactivity Disorder (Smitherman-Brown & Church, 1996). As mentioned previously, pure empirical research on the use of mandalas as a therapeutic tool is sparse. Most research into the healing aspects of mandala drawing has been limited to case studies and clinical observations (Couch, 1997; Henderson, 2007; Kellogg et al., 1977; Smitherman-Brown & Church, 1996), although they do provide promising results. Slegelis (1987) sought to examine Jung's tenet that drawing within the circular form of the mandala promotes psychological healing. More specifically, the nonverbal task of drawing mandalas would be expected to have a calming effect on their creators. Although the results of this study lend support to the argument that mandalas have calming and healing properties, the design and analyses are relatively weak and thus limit the inferences that can be drawn from the results. Curry and Kasser (2005) examined the usefulness of coloring mandalas to reduce anxiety. They assessed levels of anxiety before and after coloring of a mandala. They found that of three conditions (free-form, plaid-form and mandala drawing), individuals showed a decrease in anxiety in the mandala drawing as well as in the plaid-form condition. The control group showed no decrease in anxiety. The results demonstrated that coloring mandalas did reduce levels of clinically significant anxiety. Van Der Vennet and Serice (2013) conducted an experimental-design replication study of Curry and Kasser's (2005) research that tested whether coloring a mandala would reduce anxiety. Anxiety levels of participants were measured with the State Anxiety Inventory at the onset, after a writing exercise, and after coloring a mandala. Empirical results supported the notion that coloring a mandala reduces anxiety to a clinically significant degree as opposed to merely coloring on a blank piece of paper. Combining mandala drawing and coloring with guided imagery may result in a meditative state that helps the individual feel calm but also facilitates inner reflection and visualization (Buchalter, 2013). Coloring mandalas results in a reduction in anxiety because it allows the mind to escape from thoughts and it teaches an individual patience (Polt, 2005). Polt examined levels of depression, anxiety, energy, and concentration before and after mandala coloring. The results demonstrated that coloring mandalas did reduce levels of depression and anxiety, as well as lead to an increase in energy and concentration. Mandalas are often utilized by play therapists working within a Jungian Play Therapy orientation and by art and expressive arts therapists (Green, 2009a). In the next section, therapeutic benefits of using mandalas with an adolescent boy with ADHD are presented, through a case study.

Case Illustration

The following intervention was conducted to help facilitate treatment by offering a Jungian Play Therapy approach with an adolescent on a short-term basis (Green, Drewes & Kominski, 2013). Both the play therapist and the client were willing to try the use of the mandala. The therapist counseled the adolescent twice per week over a three-month period, which included a parent interview and subsequent family therapy sessions with the adolescent involved.

The pre-drawn mandalas were from a workbook containing 30 designs (Green, 2013). Pre-drawn mandalas were utilized for coloring purposes. During the mandala drawing session, the therapist played relaxation music from www.drericgreen.com/relaxationtunes. An original guided imagery script written by Green (2010b) was then read to the adolescent. It was adapted to include vocabulary appropriate for early adolescents and abridged slightly to be brief in duration so as to accommodate the short attention span of a typical adolescent male diagnosed with ADHD (Raffaelli et al., 2005). The script guides the listener on a metaphorical journey to the unconscious and then presents a series of central archetypes to imagine, such as the Wise Old King, the Holy Child, and Mother Earth. It concludes with instructions for creating one's own mandala including two or three symbols. During each session the therapist prefaced the reading of the script with a brief explanation and discussion of the term *archetype*.

Psychosocial and Psychopharmacological Data

Andy was a 12-year-old, seventh-grade student who was diagnosed with ADHD. Andy took 72 mg per day of Concerta medication for ADHD, had been receiving individual counseling, and participated in weekly social skills groups at his middle school. Concerta is a central nervous system stimulant prescribed to treat hyperactivity and impulse control. It has common side effects such as insomnia, aggression, and loss of appetite. Andy had excellent verbal abilities and excelled academically in math and science. He had difficulty with writing, as he reported feeling overwhelmed when reading assignments, and he experienced cognitive difficulty reducing larger assignments into smaller tasks. When presented with a multistep school project, Andy displayed disproportionate anxiety, and he remained cognitively preoccupied about the size and scope of the project. He articulated that his apprehensions centered around his thinking process of being unable to complete it. Andy had difficulty organizing his schoolwork and misplaced assignments between home and school. Despite these challenges, he maintained a B average in school.

At times, Andy presented with hypersensitivity, both emotionally and physically. He had a history of being bullied and responded by participating in self-defeating beliefs and feeling hopelessness. Andy internalized the unfair treatment by his peers. Specifically, he asked the play therapist what was wrong with him and assumed that he was at fault for his peers' mistreatment. He easily became frustrated and upset; he cried and questioned his parents, "Why did God make me this way?" A personal strength emerged from Andy's social trials: he was acutely aware of others' pain and reached out to others who were bullied or teased or whom he perceived to be emotionally hurting.

The Analytical Process of Incorporating Mandalas in Clinical Work

Throughout the play therapy process, Andy typically chose to verbally discuss issues with his therapist. However, the therapist did provide him with options to consider such as sandplay, artwork, dream work, and coloring mandalas. The client was in the position to choose when he wanted to incorporate mandalas and at what stages. The first time he elected to color a mandala started with a relaxation technique. With Andy's eyes closed, as he sat in a comfortable position, the therapist led him through a guided imagery technique for several minutes. Andy then selected a preconfigured mandala from several choices contained within Green's original workbook and created some of his own original ones in a blank circular shape (Green, 2013). The therapist instructed Andy to color the mandala. While the mandala was being colored, the therapist played nature-sounds relaxation music from www.drericgreen.com/relaxationtunes to intensify the relaxation response (Saarikallio & Erkkilä, 2007). Once the client finished coloring, the image was briefly contained (the patient contemplated the mandala in silence for 15–30 seconds). According to Allan (1988), children can benefit from drawings if the interventions provide help with individual expression and communication of the artistic creation from a phenomenological perspective. The client was then instructed to create a color key (similar to a map key) to indicate what each color on the mandala represented to him. The client was encouraged to "write the story of the mandala" on the back of the coloring page. Afterward, the therapist asked, "Is there anything you'd like to share about your mandala?" If a client does not comment, just as in sandplay, there is no mandatory or expected therapist-led verbal processing. However, some children and adolescents are verbose when it comes to explaining their unique creative activities. In that case, a therapist may choose to ask one or two of the following questions after the mandala is colored: (1) What's the story of your mandala? (2) If you were inside this mandala, what might you be feeling like? (3) What were you thinking/feeling as you were coloring this part of the mandala? and (4) How could this image relate to or remind you of a part of yourself?

Andy was interested in drawing his own mandala and quickly grasped the concept after being provided a simple overview by the therapist. He felt comfortable enough to close his eyes during the reading of the script and was able to focus through the entire script by dispelling some of his energy through moving his hands and feet while listening. At the conclusion of the reading of the script, he knew exactly what he wanted to draw. He had recently studied mythology in school and therefore was familiar with the Greek and Roman names for some of the archetypes. He drew three symbols in this order: the winged foot of Hermes, the sword and scroll of Athena, and a cross with a halo, which he labeled as the Holy Child (fig. 7.2).

Andy explained that he thought of speed and gracefulness when he thought of Hermes; and, as a runner, he identified those qualities within himself. He recognized Athena as a great scholar of wisdom and knowledge and a defender of liberty. Andy indicated his belief that he possessed the qualities of wisdom and particularly knowledge. He explained that he felt strongly about standing up for his peers' right to speak their mind in the classroom, provided they were discussing things pertinent to the lesson at the time. He expressed that it was most important for him to stand up for those students who were not "popular, rich or had famous relatives."

Andy labeled the cross and halo as the *Holy Child* but discussed it as "a Redeemer, Forgiver, and the Savior." He explained that he felt that he was good at forgiving people and that when faced with peers saying or doing unkind things to him he chose to "try to let it go and say to [himself], 'they don't know what they're doing' and to forgive them, too." He lamented, "It is very rare that I meet people who actually care about who *I* am instead of caring if I'm popular, or rich or have famous relatives." He then went on to share how his own experiences have helped him to develop empathy and awareness of instances when other people are hurting but try to conceal the hurt with false displays of happiness. Andy recounted a particular in- cident with a fellow student who had said someone he "really loved" had died. Andy became teary as he explained, "I felt sad for [him] and actually almost started to cry." He briefly discussed how he had tried to comfort the classmate. The play therapist used *amplification*, a Jungian intervention that entails helping a client carry forward images and symbols to further delve into their meaning through artistic means (Green, 2012b). The therapist suggested that he draw a symbol for this, and Andy drew a series of inter- connected hearts to symbolize the "love that kept growing and growing"

Figure 7.2. "Holy Child" mandala

in the family. Andy appeared to feel soothed by creating and coloring the symbol, as evidenced by his relaxed shoulder stance and facial muscles.

During the second session of coloring mandalas, Andy selected a design of a series of overlapping circles, which created seven overlapping flower-type designs with six petals each. Fincher (2000) identifies this as a Hindu design representing Creation from the Great Round stage of Crystallization, "a time of fulfillment, satisfaction, and completion" (p. 14). Andy did not see this caption.

Initially, Andy spoke a lot; and although he continued coloring, he was frequently distracted by various stimuli, including the names of the colors and Spanish translations of words printed on the crayons. After a few minutes of quiet coloring, he began to talk about something in his life that was causing him anxiety: the change in the family's usual summer vacation to attend a family wedding. He began to color inward within his boundaries of the inner mandala he had created. He shifted the topic of conversation back to the crayon colors as he switched to color between the inner and outer mandalas. He worked in circular motions throughout the course of the task, turning the paper in circles as he worked, and became quiet. He remained quiet until he became anxious after accidentally coloring a small portion of the drawing a color he hadn't intended; at that time he tensed his shoulders and spoke to express his frustration and disappointment. The therapist acknowledged his intent and reflected his feelings. He relaxed his shoulders and switched to another dialogue about the crayon colors before trailing off and returning to work silently for several moments.

He made conventional color choices for the sun, sky, clouds, and grass but unconventional choices for the gold stem, silver buds, and brown petals (fig. 7.3). Andy titled his mandala "the flower of life." In describing the story of the mandala, he told a creation story, starting with "let there be light" from a divine figure that he also described as "the hope that keeps you going." He went on to describe (a) the grass as a "life bearer" for the flower of life (i.e., a *Mother Earth* reference), (b) the sky as a space where birds could fly freely or the sea floating on itself (i.e., possibly a reference to the dividing of the waters into sky and sea in the Judeo-Christian Creation story), (c) the stem of the flower as akin to the golden horn of a newborn unicorn, to him signifying birth (i.e., the *Divine Child*), (d) the silver bud of the flower as like the silver horn of a mature unicorn (i.e., the *Animus* or masculine archetype), and (e) the brown of the flower as "the soul, the part of you that even when you die it won't" (i.e., this may represent the *Self* archetype). Andy colored his soul brown. Allan (1988) suggests that the use of brown in children's drawings often signifies "inhibitions, repression, and depression" (p. 148). Yet, when the therapist asked how he would feel if he were in this picture, Andy said he would feel "pretty happy" and even indicated where he would lie on the grass in the picture. At the end of the session, Andy spoke about the brown petals again and said they were brown like the dirt that "has the nutrients for you to keep you going" and said cheerfully that brown was a beautiful color for a flower.

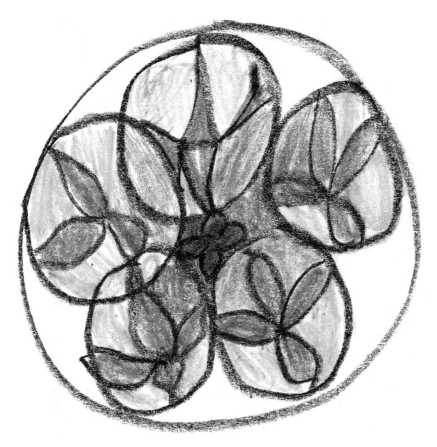

Figure 7.3. "Flower of Life" mandala

Post-Analysis

As a survivor of bullying and a student with special needs, Andy often dwelled on his social challenges to connect with other peers and his minor academic shortcomings. Creating his own mandala encouraged self-healing, promoted development of the Self, and provided Andy with an opportunity to recognize and appreciate his positive qualities such as speed, grace, wisdom, mercy, and righteousness. Andy's colored "Creation" mandala was replete with representations and references to archetypes from the collective unconscious; it is unlikely that traditional talk therapy would have brought forth this amount of symbolic information. Both drawing and coloring mandalas allowed Andy to externalize personal images in a visual medium. This visual representation created a bridge that allowed him to become aware of his internal strengths and verbally process abstractions with the therapist. Immediate benefits were observed by the therapist: the client was able to relax during the mandala coloring and, with the aid of a guided imagery meditation, could elicit personal symbols and metaphors regarding his life. Andy reported that the process of creating the mandalas and the personal interpretation of them helped him to gain access to and underscore personal strengths. The therapeutic outcome at the termination of psycho-therapy was positive, as the adolescent self-reported feeling less stress and being more emotionally available to communicate with those around him, especially his peers. The therapist also advocated for the client at his school for a safer emotional and physical environment from the bullying that was occurring.

Clinical Implications for Play Therapists

Coloring mandalas with adolescent males with ADHD within a Jung-ian Play Therapy framework may provide access to self-healing through its meditative process. Play therapists planning to incorporate mandalas into individual therapy with adolescents should consider several factors in order to provide the greatest benefits. To familiarize the client with the concept of mandalas, it is generally considered more facilitative to ask clients to color pre-drawn mandalas before creating their own, so that they have a tangible contextualization from which to build upon (Cox & Cohen, 2000). Second, play therapists may want to provide a brief overview of archetypes, as the author did at the beginning of this chapter. Adolescents understand what symbols are, but they may not be familiar with the term *archetypes*. However, this is not cogent, since the term *archetype* can be removed from the guided imagery exercise and replaced with the word *symbol*. Third, play therapists need to engage in continuous psycho-diagnostic assessment to evaluate their client's abilities. Clients do not need to be able to consciously interpret their mandalas to benefit from coloring them; the emergence of the *self-healing archetype* is what heals (Baggerly & Green, 2013; Green, 2009b). However, drawing mandalas does require some abstracting ability; therefore, therapists should consider their client's abstract reasoning abilities in order to avoid or limit psychological frustration.

The play therapist should acquire training in basic art therapy principles to understand the expressive art therapy intervention's rationale, utility, and healing potential within the psychotherapeutic context. Also, play therapists should seek professional development and training in guided imagery before using it as a conduit to expressive art therapy interventions. Therapists must ethically practice only within their scope of supervised training and education, especially play therapists seeking to incorporate tenets from the expressive art therapy modalities (Green & Drewes, 2013). Moreover, play therapists must receive specialized training in Jungian Play Therapy and interpretation before attempting to integrate these types of specialized treatment approaches. Fourth, play therapists should change activities when necessary. The mandala drawing activity requires concentration. If the client seems tired or distracted, a clinician may choose another expressive art therapy activity that the adolescent responds to within the clinical setting. Finally, play therapists should affirm the adolescent's effort. Adolescents may feel uncertain about their abilities when trying a new activity. Affirming the adolescent's effort and acknowledging his commitment to the therapeutic process may improve the therapeutic relationship and encourage the emergence of the self-healing properties in play therapy to emerge and be fully realized. And as with all other Jungian interventions, play therapists must be engaged in ongoing personal analysis or supervision so that they can continuously work on their own issues and counter-transferences and avoid contaminating the consulting room.

8

With Bereaved Children

We can't change a thing until we first learn to accept it.

—Carl Jung

———

Family sand tray (FST) with bereaved clients, especially young children, may assist family members in communicating their intrapersonal world of grief through symbolic methods. Specifically, play therapists using FST provide the opportunity for children to share feelings with caretakers that may be developmentally difficult to verbalize. With FST, children use nonthreatening images to portray feelings and struggles associated with the death of a loved one. The focus of this chapter is the importance of including caretakers and family members in bereaved children's sandplay. A clinical vignette illuminates the potential benefits of incorporating FST with bereaved children. The chapter concludes with implications for Jungian play therapists.

Loss is a prevalent component of children's lives; one in seven children under the age of 10 encounters the death of a caretaker or loved one (Batts, 2004). Contemporary authors (Barth, 2006; Crenshaw, 2005; Stroebe & Schut, 2001; Webb, 2002) have emphasized the potential for adverse psychosocial effects upon bereaved children who may be emotionally unable to resolve grief as effectively as an older adolescent or adult. Because children sometimes have difficulties verbalizing their thoughts, feelings, and needs, it is necessary that play therapists develop an understanding of the developmental context of grief in children. Additionally, it is important to use effective counseling strategies to meet bereaved children's mental health needs (Gil, 2006).

Grief is a process rather than a specific emotion like sadness or fear, and these reactions to loss can occur as feelings, physical sensations, cognitions, and disordered behaviors in children. Bowlby (1960) defined grief as "the sequence of subjective states that follow loss and accompany mourning" (p. 11). Children experience loss and mourn the death of loved ones, including peers, parents, grandparents, caregivers, and pets. The impact of a significant grief experience may negatively alter a child's perception of the world. She may begin to view the world as an unstable, uncertain environment (Busch & Kimble, 2001).

In the following sections of the chapter, the developmental context of children's grief and the importance of a therapeutic relationship are examined. Factors that influence bereaved children's engagement in play therapy are also addressed. The rationale for play therapy with bereaved children is presented with a focus on family sandplay therapy (FST). The inclusion of significant caretakers or family members in bereaved children's sand therapy may be a vital component of healing as it provides a familial context. The process, content, and outcomes of FST with a bereaved child are illustrated in a case study. Finally, implications for Jungian play therapists are provided.

The Developmental Context of Children's Grief

Young children's (a) understanding of the concept of death, (b) availability of and access to coping mechanisms, and (c) grief-specific factors are affected by their developmental stage and contextual influences (Oltjenbruns, 2001; Shapiro, 1994). Cognizance of the stages of natural childhood development provides a foundation for understanding children's varied responses to loss. This depth of knowledge augments clinicians' insight into the childhood bereavement process and potential play themes evidenced during the psychotherapeutic process. Children's chronological conceptualizations of death are illustrated in table 8.1. These conceptualizations should be viewed by readers as fluid and often circular. The age groups are nonrestrictive; they represent developmental stages in which bereaved children's understandings of death and play behaviors overlap (Busch & Kimble, 2001).

Children have a limited repertoire of coping strategies, compared to the adaptive capabilities of adults. Because of their young age, they may have

Table 8.1. The developmental and therapeutic context of children's grief

Ages	Conceptualization of death	Possible themes evidenced in play therapy sessions	Implications for bereavement
2–5	Sees death as reversible or temporary Displays magical thinking (i.e., wishes someone dead, or deceased person returns) Is aware of changes in routine but unable to attribute them to death in the family	Reflects sadness, confusion, guilt, aggression during play Portrays death-related magical thinking through toys (e.g., mother returns after leaving house repeatedly) Regresses to earlier developmental behavior (shown directly or through toys) Buries toys Loses and relocates toys purposefully during session Expresses grief in artwork, covering bright colors with dark colors (i.e., draws house then paints page dark color, declaring it's nighttime)	Has self-blame issues Uses concrete language and magical thinking to understand causality May understand adult explanations of cause of death in concrete and self-blame language
5–9	Gradually comprehends death as permanent and final Retains some magical thinking	May reflect guilt, anger, aggression, chaos, regression, or compulsive caregiving during play May welcome use of creative arts and sand because of difficulty expressing feelings verbally Buries toys Personifies death during play (e.g., monster takes dead person away) May show need to experience omnipotence and power during play Displays fantasies about deceased person	May have concrete understanding of cause of death, but confusion is likely May appear unaffected and have deliberate illusion that deceased person is present May feel shame because of differences compared to intact families

Table 8.1. cont.

Ages	Conceptualization of death	Possible themes evidenced in play therapy sessions	Implications for bereavement
9–13	Is cognitively aware of death's finality Has difficulty conceiving own death or that of a loved one Reasons concretely about how and why death occurs	May reflect anger, guilt, possessiveness, or aggression in play May show defiance to play therapist or through symbols portrayed in play Buries toys	Remains vulnerable to constructing fantasies that deceased family member may return May entangle grief and loss with separation issues

Source: Adapted from Busch & Kimble, 2001; Glazer & Clark, 1999; Mauk & Sharpnack, 2006; Shapiro, 1994; Webb, 2002.

narrow experiences related to loss, particularly as compared to adults. Unlike adults, bereaved children typically experience inadequate comfort from verbal condolences. Likewise, children often do not have the linguistic capacity to describe emotions or their internal preoccupations. Instead, children often communicate with others in behavioral or symbolic ways, such as through artwork and playing with toys (Aldwin, 1994; Moody & Moody, 1991; Oltjenbruns, 2001). Children's grief may appear more sporadic and short-lived; however, their limited verbal communication skills may mask the duration of their grief (Mauk & Sharpnack, 2006).

Webb (2002) noted additional discriminations between the grief reactions of children and adults: (a) some children have a limited capacity to tolerate emotional pain; (b) children may have an increased socialized sensitivity regarding being different from their nongrieving peers; and (c) some children are incapable of formulating a cognitive appraisal to understand the implications of death, such as irreversibility, universality, and inevitability. According to Doka (2000) and Speece and Brent (1996), children's grief experiences may be affected by their understanding of: (a) universality (i.e., all things must eventually die, and one cannot avoid death); (b) irreversibility (i.e., once something dies, it cannot become alive again); (c) nonfunctionality (i.e., once something dies, it ceases to be able to engage in life-related behaviors); and (d) causality (i.e., understanding the causes of death). It is important to recognize that cognitive developmental age rather than chronological age is the primary influence on the conceptualization and understanding of death.

Although children's cognitive understanding of death is often presented in linear age-specific categories (table 8.1), the impact of death may affect children throughout personal, social, and emotional domains. Moreover, their cognitive appraisal or interpretation of death may be inconsistent with their level of maturity and may differ according to life experiences encompassing the death of a loved one. Issues of bereavement are interlaced with those of development. As children mature, they typically resolve the experience of death differently than in their earlier years (Miller, 1995; Oltjenbruns, 2001; Silverman, 2000). Thus, one goal of bereavement intervention for children is establishing a developmentally appropriate and supportive environment, in which children can continue toward mastery of tasks crucial to each developmental stage (Wolfe & Senta, 1995).

Moderating Grief Factors

In addition to the developmental context of children's grief experiences, moderating factors exist that influence their adaptive or maladaptive grieving processes. Moderating factors, or lack thereof, can be crucial in determining the necessity of an outside referral for a child or family following the death of a loved one (Melvin & Lukeman, 2000). A dynamic interaction exists between potential vulnerabilities for psychological difficulties and protective factors (Mauk & Sharpnack, 2006). Individual factors affecting the construction of a child's grief experience include the child's age, developmental stage, cognitive-processing ability, temperament, access to coping and adjustment resources, and past experience with loss. Death-related factors, such as whether the death was anticipated, the degree of pain, the cultural elements of stigma, the child's expression of closure, and the meaning of the loss as indicated by the child's relationship to the deceased, all affect the course of bereavement for the child (Goldman, 2001; Stroebe & Schut, 2001; Webb, 2002).

The quality and number of supportive relationships play a seminal role in a child's positive adjustment. How a child responds to death is often mediated by how the family members, especially significant caretakers, react to the loss. For example, factors such as family cohesiveness, psychosocial family stressors, the family style of coping, and family messages about how to display grief often influence the child's grief reaction (Shapiro, 1994; Webb, 2002). Family issues such as incongruence, interpersonal discord, emotional unavailability of caregivers, and instability may contribute to a bereaved child's referral to psychotherapy. Effective counseling approaches for bereaved children and their families are described in subsequent sections, based upon the aforementioned mediating factors that compromise children's ability to cope with grief.

Expressive Therapies for Bereaved Children and Their Families

Play Therapy

Developing a counseling relationship in which a child feels understood and free to communicate his innermost yearnings, fears, and wishes is often more complex than beginning a counseling relationship with adults (Fiorini & Mullen, 2006). Therefore, it is important to guide children's natural efforts to communicate their loss at the beginning of the therapeutic relationship with creative methods tailored to meet their developmental needs. Communication with children is unique. Toys provide a language that enables the counselor to connect to and understand the child (Rotter & Bush, 2000; Way & Bremner, 2005).

Therapeutic powers inherent in play with bereaved children include (a) communication of the loss through toys, symbols, and images in nonthreatening ways; (b) psycho-educational components of death; (c) abreaction of powerful emotions via metaphorical play; and (d) rapport-building to foster a nonjudgmental, therapeutic dyad in which the child feels safe to make sense of loss and develop coping strategies (Reddy et al., 2005).

The expression and acceptance of sad or confused emotions, often through play, enables a child to develop a personal understanding of the loss (Ayyash-Abdo, 2001; Webb, 2000). The play therapist patiently witnesses the child's emerging grief reactions. The child leads the grief work, because the therapist believes the child is capable of self-direction and healing; the therapist does not evaluate the child's grief reactions. In the therapeutic context, therefore, play therapy offers the unconditional acceptance needed by children who have not sufficiently mourned the loss of a loved one so they can proceed with their lives (Carroll, 1995).

Research on Play Therapy with Bereaved Children

Despite the scarcity of empirical evidence on the effectiveness of play therapy with bereaved children, several case studies have provided anecdotal support that play media, such as sand, may help address issues associated with grief in children. Authors have indicated that sand therapy may help to decrease (a) irritability, (b) social withdrawal, (c) hypersomnia or insomnia, and (d) perceived guilt (Carey, 1990; Carroll, 1995; Glazer & Clark, 1999; Green & Ironside, 2004; Webb, 2002, 2003).

Jungian Sandplay Therapy versus (the Generic) Sand Tray Therapy

The crux of sandplay is that a therapist witnesses the sandplay process respectfully, honors the psyche, and focuses on the depth and meaning in the symbols and the client's psyche's relationship to them. The therapeutic rationale for sandplay is linked to the notion that all therapy is grief work (Preston-Dillon, 2007). The counselor provides the *free and protected space* in which a creation in the sand may symbolize the inner world of grief and the healing potential of the client's psyche (Kalff, 1980). The *protected space* refers to the way the therapist listens, observes, and nonjudgmentally accepts the emotional content that becomes activated by the sand therapy process (McNulty, 2007). There is an emphasis on activating the self-healing force in a child's psyche so that the child may resolve psychosocial struggles (Allan & Berry, 1987; Allan & Brown, 1993). The emerging pictures in the tray illustrate the unconscious conflicts of the client as sand therapy provides an opportunity for both symbolic and realistic *grounding* to occur. Sand tray therapy is a generic, theory-based approach that involves therapist interaction within the sand scene and more directed interventions.

Authors have cited several therapeutic benefits resulting from sandplay therapy (Allan & Berry, 1987; Boik & Goodwin, 2000; Goldman, 2001; Green & Ironside, 2004). First, sandplay frees creativity, perceptions, feelings, and memories as the client transports unconscious thoughts and feelings from the interior to the exterior realm of consciousness. Second, many children view sandplay as a natural form of expression, and they are readily drawn to it. Although some children and adults seem reluctant to draw or paint, they tend to respond positively to sandplay because they feel free to create with less self-criticism or constraint. Furthermore, because sandplay involves nonverbal expression, it engenders a necessary therapeutic distance from distressing or traumatic events for clients.

Sandplay is distinguished from sand tray therapy because it permits the child to create a sand picture that provides concrete images of thoughts and feelings. Also, sandplay provides a unique kinesthetic quality, as the extremely tactile experience of manipulating sand can be a therapeutic encounter; touching and playing in the sand may produce a calming effect in anxious children. From a Jungian perspective, the primary therapeutic benefit of sandplay involves the healing power of the client's psyche represented by symbols witnessed by the therapist through an honoring of depth and meaning. Kalff (1980) emphasized that the transformative experience of creating a picture in the sand contains the healing. Sandplay may facilitate healing and transformation by releasing conflicts from the unconscious in symbolic form and by supporting a healthy reordering of psychological contents (Turner, 2005).

Sandplay with Bereaved Children

The rationale for sandplay with bereaved children is multifaceted. First, a sand tray and figurines can be mechanisms for a child to express affect while a therapist witnesses the child's phenomenological experience of grief (Fry, 2000; Preston-Dillon, 2007). It is in the showing, rather than the telling, that children can explore their conceptualizations of life, death, dying, grieving, and surviving. During the session emotional healing is emphasized, helping children restore conscious awareness of the past. Thereby the process of necessary grief is realized. The process of sandplay provides opportunities for children to (a) express loss; (b) say goodbye; (c) allow for continued grief as it changes over time; (d) remember, reflect, and reintegrate; (e) feel anchored as they make the loss tangible by providing a space of contact to physically touch the loss; and (f) share their view of the situation.

Family Sand Tray Therapy (FST)

Because development and coping capacities occur typically within a familial context, play therapists should include family members in treatment planning with bereaved children as stipulated through the systems theory paradigm (Fox, 2006; Shapiro, 1994). Integrating components of systems theory and Jungian sandplay, play therapists focus on the family as a monolithic unit—rather than limiting focus to the individuals within the system. When approaching play therapy from a systems perspective, the clinician includes the broader context of the child and the goal of bolstering the network of interpersonal relationships among family members (Anderson, 1993; Carey, 2006b; Gil, 1994, 2003). Because sandplay is strictly individual work, the use of groups and families in sand is always referred to as sand tray.

FST, when paired within a systemic lens, is based on the premise that stimuli affecting one family member must affect all members because of the depth of connective qualities of familial relationships (Carey, 1999). Each member of the family experiencing bereavement will have an impact on the other family members collectively. The play therapist understands the impact of the loss on the family system and that the coping strategies available within the family context shape the treatment plan (Bailey, 2000; Crenshaw, 2005). Family systems concepts provide therapists with a dynamic model for empowering individuals and families to heal as they grieve through the process of sand tray (Shapiro, 1994; Silverman, 2000).

Process and Procedures

During the intake before play therapists devise treatment plans for bereaved children, they should obtain information regarding (a) how the family system is organized; (b) how various roles are assigned; and (c) distinctive characteristics including family boundaries, patterns of communication, the family as a problem-solving unit, and styles of coping. Additionally, a clinician must examine the aspects of family life that are disrupted by death and the mechanisms that families rely upon to reestablish the stabilizing structures that support their normative functioning (Silverman, 2000).

The child typically participates in individual play therapy sessions for a couple of weeks before the play therapist uses FST in treatment. Therapists should be cautious when using FST if the level of trust within a group is compromised (Pearson & Wilson, 2001) or if the child has not yet been involved in individual sand sessions. Once the play therapist has decided to include FST in therapy, the therapist needs to provide a brief and developmentally appropriate introduction to FST and prepare the family for the upcoming session. The therapist needs to emphasize that sand therapy is a medium used to address a variety of issues related to grieving. The therapist should provide information about boundaries, limits, and safety (Carey, 1999).

During the first FST session, all family members should agree upon boundaries and guidelines that create an emotionally safe, therapeutic environment for all persons involved (Pearson & Wilson, 2001). This session should include an orientation to the playroom. The therapist then explains that family members are free to use whatever figurines they choose to create a picture in the sand tray. It is their picture; therefore there is no *right* or *wrong*. After these directions are given, the play therapist emphasizes the opportunity at the end of the session for family members to (a) share observations, (b) tell a story about their world, and (c) share what their world might represent to others (Carey, 2006b). After the explanation and answering of questions, the family begins to choose figurines and create their picture in the sand tray. If resistance to play is displayed by adults, it important for the therapist to encourage them to remember what it was like to play as a child and to emphasize the importance of play for both adult and child well-being (Botkin, 2000). The therapist should not only seek to create a safe therapeutic context for children, but also for adults (Lund et al., 2002).

During every session utilizing FST, the therapist observes the process of how the family begins and proceeds with the task of creating a picture in the sand. When observing family dynamics, the therapist notices the roles of the family members (Boik & Goodwin, 2000). The therapist may gain insight into family alliances by observing the choices made, such as who chooses to work together, the figurines that are selected, and leaders in the selection process (Carey, 1991, 1994). Using a broader lens, play therapists can obtain useful information about the family by observing (a) their ability and willingness to organize and complete a task; (b) metaphors created by the family; (c) the level of contact and emotional connectedness; (d) the level of insight; (e) caretaker intrusion, control, affect, praise, communication, and use of threats; and (f) boundaries, communication styles, family cohesion, and rigidity (Gil, 2003; Gil & Sobol, 2000; Landreth, 2001). While a family creates a picture in the sand, the therapist observes whether members argue or cooperate and whether one person seems to overrule others. Also, the therapist takes note of whether the family talks or works silently and the level of participation of each member, as this may provide context to family interaction patterns.

To conclude every FST session, post-scene discussion is used. The play therapist gives each family member an opportunity to tell a story about what she or he contributed to the picture in the sand tray. This discussion may be valuable to a therapist as it assists in consolidating observations and perspectives on the session (Carey, 2006b). The content of what is verbalized and also what is suggested through symbol, metaphor, and metaphoric language are important to understand family dynamics (Gil & Sobol, 2000). However, the therapist should offer a minimum amount of interpretation until the family structure is strengthened. The therapist can become more directive and choose who should work together during subsequent sessions, perhaps pairing family members who are experiencing particular issues that need to be addressed. Finally, FST is an inclusive experience, because it honors the developmental level of the family and offers the opportunity for self-expression (Homeyer & Sweeney, 2005). Families working together on sand trays may gain insights about their dynamics as the activity opens broader communication within the family and actively engages all family members in the group healing process.

Rationale and Benefits of FST with Bereaved Children

There are several reasons cited for including caretakers in a bereaved child's sand work (Bailey & Sori, 2000; Dermer et al., 2006). Caretakers know valuable and intimate information about their child. Including caretakers in FST can help them to provide support and encouragement to assist their grieving child. Furthermore, including caretakers in bereaved children's sand tray allows the therapist to observe caretaker-child dynamics during the sessions. The goal of FST is for caretakers to help their child create an experience that encourages the communication of understanding and respect. Therapeutic change occurs more rapidly in bereaved children if family members are included in the process and become agents of change themselves (Boik & Goodwin, 2000; LeBlanc & Ritchie, 1999).

Case Illustration

When Michael was 6 years old, his father, Norman, entered a residential rehabilitation center for individuals with heroin addiction. As a result of drug relapses over two years, Norman vacillated from the rehabilitation center to his home, where he lived with Michael's biological mother, Kathleen. Because of the marital strain, Kathleen had filed for separation. Because of financial restraints and the distance between the center and home, Kathleen could not visit Norman. Norman died of an unexpected heart attack while staying at a treatment center. The coroner reported that the death stemmed from a drug overdose.

During the intake, approximately two months after Norman died, Kathleen described Michael's presenting problems as psychosocial difficulties related to grief. She described diminished self-esteem, disordered behaviors such as not going to sleep at a specified hour, boundary problems, perfectionism as illustrated through Michael's insistence on making straight As, and separation anxiety. The boundary and separation issues were evidenced through Michael's unwillingness to spend the night away from Kathleen after his father's death. She was also concerned because Michael had slept in her bed since Norman moved away for treatment.

The therapist initiated the work with an extended developmental assessment (Gil, 2006) that lasted approximately three sessions. The therapist created a behavioral treatment plan, which included expressive therapies. In the eleventh session, the therapist asked Michael to create a picture in the sand tray. Michael appeared excited or happy as he began to create his picture. He smiled and approached the activity with interest. He seemed proud of his picture as shown through his numerous comments about liking the way it appeared.

His first picture exemplified a theme of aggression, since he created a war scene. Most of the people figurines carried weapons. Michael often made shooting sounds and motions as he placed the figurines in the tray. A motion theme was also present in Michael's first sand tray, as indicated through figurine choice and placement. The presence of 11 vehicles, a horse, weaponry, a waterway, and two bridges suggested movement. The movement and repositioning of figurines during the construction of the sand picture supported the theme of motion (Turner, 2005). Throughout the session he counted the number of soldiers and vehicles on each side of the war and made several comments about wanting it to be fair. Michael included several figurines that represented helping functions, such as a fire truck, a police car, and an ambulance.

During the first post-scene discussion, Michael's desire to be understood was evident as he explained his picture and corrected the therapist's responses if they did not match what he was conveying. Michael expressed a desire to be on the rescue crew and away from the fighting, aligning with his mother's previous description that Michael's personality matched closely one who protects.

During subsequent counseling sessions, Michael more freely talked about his father and the impact of his death, but he resisted discussing his current living situation with his mother. After four individual counseling sessions with Michael, the therapist incorporated FST into counseling so that Michael and his mother could express feelings related to their grief. The play therapist prepared them for the next session by discussing boundaries and guidelines regarding FST.

At the beginning of the sixth session, Michael and Kathleen were invited to the sand tray and were instructed to use any of the figurines to silently construct a picture in the sand. The therapist emphasized that there was no *right* or *wrong* way to create picture. He further explained that he would give them an opportunity to discuss the sand scene when the picture seemed complete.

Initially, Michael and Kathleen sanded together for approximately five minutes. Then Michael worked for 15 minutes as his mother observed. The completed world included trees, bridges, fenced-in sharks, pirates attacking praying children, ambulances, two sharks, and a joker placed on the upper left corner edge of the tray with a menacing pirate nearby. As compared to the time when Michael created his individual sand scene, he seemed more anxious. He was reluctant to make direct eye contact with the therapist or his mother. Additionally, he fidgeted with his fingers in a nervous manner. He was reluctant to engage in post-scene discussion.

Notable family dynamics within this first family session included Kathleen's dissatisfaction (i.e., "We can't do this," "How much more do you really need," and "We can't really put praying children outside") and her attempt to control Michael's choices and time in creating the scene. Kathleen seemed to feel discomfort or resistance as she waited for her son to finish. For example, she frequently sighed, and she attempted multiple unrelated conversations with the therapist while Michael was sanding. Michael commented that he felt like the joker, and Kathleen laughed at that comment.

The process of creating this family sand scene provided important information on family dynamics that had not previously been revealed through other aspects of counseling. For example, Kathleen appeared to want more parental control, and she was uncomfortable talking about Norman. Kathleen had difficulty understanding and responding to Michael's feelings. Michael revealed the self-image of the joker, possibly constructed to work through his current emotional pain in nonthreatening ways. Michael's identification with the joker is noteworthy because the joker is generally thought of as a symbol for humor and fun. However this joker was fighting with a pirate. Michael's comment on feeling like he was the joker is also of great interest because of his teacher's description of Michael's clownlike behaviors in school.

In a subsequent FST session, the therapist asked Michael to create a picture depicting his mother's feelings. Michael sanded a scene of soldiers circling around a mother figure. A boy figure was on the outside of the circle of soldiers and was facing the mother. When asked to comment on the scene, Michael stated sullenly, "The mother is running from the house because the boy is acting crazy, and the boy does not want her to be killed and is trying to get her back." Then Michael buried the figurines beneath the sand and became quiet.

Later during the same FST session, Kathleen was asked to create a picture illustrating how Michael felt. Kathleen chose figurines to represent sports in which Michael participated before Norman's death. She included a figurine to represent herself and Norman. After Kathleen commented on the elements of her scene, Michael began to share a story about his father. In the story Norman sent Michael a talking picture frame with an old picture of them after Michael's soccer team had won a game. Norman said, "I'm proud of you son." Kathleen stated angrily that Norman was never proud of anything but his drug-usage, and she changed the topic abruptly.

Michael responded by burying the figurines in his mother's sand scene. This may have symbolized Michael's desire to bury his pain and hurt associated with his desire to be heard and understood by his mother. The therapist acknowledged Michael's feelings of grief and remembering, which he had been reluctant to express previously, and invited Kathleen to respond to Michael's feelings. She was able to respond to Michael and acknowledged her difficulty with talking about his father. She stated that she did not want to be emotionally vulnerable.

During a later FST session, the therapist asked Michael and his mother to create a picture together to represent their family. Michael chose figurines that he said were his cousins and uncle. He did not choose figurines to represent himself, Kathleen, or Norman. He enacted a crashing scene between jets taking off. Michael appeared unwilling or unable to compose his family perhaps because he was still grappling with Norman's death. After Kathleen explained her contributions to the scene, which included Michael as the joker, a mother figurine to represent herself, and a father figurine to represent Norman, Michael began to bury the figurines without speaking. From a Jungian viewpoint, this may have represented Michael's psyche attempting to heal itself by burying the pain of this father's loss and his mother's compromised emotional support.

Over the next three months, Michael's ability to freely talk with Kathleen about Norman's death improved. A theme of his need to protect his mother continued to emerge. As Kathleen began to understand her son and his needs, and cope with her own feelings toward Norman's death, she started to become more emotionally available for her son. Michael returned to sleeping in his own bed. Although he still struggled with academic issues at school, such as perfectionism with his grades, he did begin to alter his role as the class clown. His teachers stated that he became integrated with the rest of his peers and curtailed many of his attention-seeking behaviors.

Conclusion

Throughout the family sand tray process, Michael and his mother participated in self-healing and symbolically expressed grief that was otherwise challenging to express verbally. Denial, role confusion, guilt, and anger were developmental aspects of grief that were addressed throughout the FST process. Michael expressed his guilt and anger as shown through his sand scene with the mother figure fleeing from the house, with no father figure present, because of the boy who was acting like he was crazy. Michael's need to protect his mother was addressed as he felt more comfortable disclosing details about his deceased father during FST. Michael exhibited maturational achievement as he began to sleep apart from his mother comfortably in his own bed. Kathleen's ability to place her son's feelings before her own and realize her effect on her son's healing made it possible for the family to move forward.

Implications for Jungian Play Therapists

Jungian play therapists must recognize and respect that all children view death differently. No one method of treating issues related to bereavement is accepted universally. What is most important is listening and adapting the treatment to meet the child where he is developmentally (Barth, 2006). As play therapists incorporate family work in sand sessions, they may bring hope and healing to grieving families. FST does have the potential to be a powerful tool in working within a family unit as depth is honored. Family sand tray can be a powerful expressive therapy with bereaved children and offers a context for grieving during the therapeutic process.

The case study illustrates the value of family sand tray therapy in helping a child during the grieving process. It is imperative that play therapists be informed of the developmental context of grief and indications of problems during the grieving process so that they can better assess a bereaved child's need for counseling and also answer caretakers' questions about the typical grieving experiences of children. Furthermore, play therapists can collaborate with local grief centers with regard to trainings on grief issues in children and resources for psychotherapy for families in need. Play therapists who have a background in family therapy need to participate in training before deeming themselves qualified to incorporate families in play therapy. It is germane for play therapists to consider a systems approach when working with bereaved children and incorporate significant caretakers or family members to help children overcome psychological barriers to successful adaptation following the loss of a loved one.

9

With a Child Who Is Diagnosed with Autism

You meet your destiny on the very road you take to avoid it.

—Carl Jung

———

This chapter provides an overview of the theoretical and research support of using Jungian Play Therapy with children affected by autism, but only within a comprehensive, multi-disciplinary team of highly qualified mental health and educational experts. Interpretation and analysis are covered in detail as techniques to use with this special population. Finally, a case study is presented with a child diagnosed with Asperger's and receiving Jungian Play Therapy treatment.

According to Shunsen (2010), Jungian sandplay therapy mediates some of the language barriers of children with autism, stimulates problem-solving through simulations in the sand, emphasizes the development of self-reliance and self-control ability via the principles of natural teaching, and improves their imagination and creativeness. In a 10-week school-based action research study with children with autism, Lu, Peterson, Lacroix, and Rousseau (2010) found that sandplay increased verbal expression and symbolic play and improved children's sustained social interaction. The authors concluded that creativity-based interventions, such as Jungian sandplay, provide a complementary approach alongside behavioral models when counseling children with autism. However, substantial research needs to be undertaken before conclusions of efficacy can be made regarding Jungian play's effectiveness with children with Asperger's.

The theoretical support for utilizing Jungian play is that children with Asperger Syndrome have the capacity to communicate verbally, a core requirement for the analytical process. Liu, Shih, and Ma (2011) described how children with Asperger Syndrome scored equal to and often superior to their typically developing peers in areas of creativity and originality. Jungian Play Therapy incorporates symbol work, which requires the child to use creative and original play within the psychotherapy. Therefore, children with Asperger Syndrome (AS) may find Jungian play to be appealing and complementary to their attributes and strengths, which may promote self-motivation to resolve psychosocial difficulties.

Temple Grandin (2006) observes that many high-functioning children with AS view the world in pictures or images, and they make sense of external stimuli through visual thinking. This view would be complementary to the analytical premise that symbols and images created in drawings, read about in myths, and enacted in sandplay are integral to a child's psychological growth. Grandin, herself a leading voice and doctoral scholar with autism, comments: "Every problem I've ever solved started with my ability to visualize and see the world in pictures" (p. 4). Her views are substantiated by research demonstrating that many high-functioning children with autism score at least as highly as their typically developing peers in visuoperceptual processing (Bertrone et al., 2005; Caron et al., 2004).

The term *analysis*, from Jungian *analytical* Play Therapy, refers to reducing complexes into taut, understandable components through visual means. In play therapy with children, analysis means listening to and observing a child to elucidate the complexes that are creating anomalies and need mediation to reduce stress and make meaning out of psychosocial difficulties. Many children with AS rely heavily upon the left-brain hemispheric section, where analytical processing occurs, as opposed to right-brain intuiting and emoting (Rosenn, 2009). So from this viewpoint, Jungian Play Therapy may be beneficial to children with AS because the therapist may be able to more easily empathize with the child's disparate inner world that is sometimes emotionally flat and monotonous, as children with AS may place considerable passion into analytical, rule-based activities (Grandin, 2006). Jungian analyst Michael Fordham illustrates this concept in his book *The Self and Autism* (1976), as he provides anecdotal support from his various clinical cases when using Jungian child analysis with high-functioning children with autism.

Daniel Rosenn (2009), a medical doctor and expert on Asperger Syndrome, commented on the inherent difficulties but the importance of incorporating insight-based psychotherapy (in contrast to CBT) with children with Asperger Syndrome:

> After a great deal of tactful and thoughtful effort on the therapist's part, the patient experiences deeply emotional insights or self-revelations, and these presumably lead to internal change and adaptation. These also are very hard to harvest in Asperger's, where most therapy is cognitive behavioral, and relies on patterning of external behaviors and actions. If you are the kind of therapist who searches for these moments of affective transcendency, it can be like panning for gold nuggets in a muddy Sacramento River. Insight-oriented psychotherapy can be very lonely and empty. There are many adults and even older children with Asperger's, with whom one can do satisfying humanistic-relational therapy. (p. 7)

Readers are advised to continue to survey the most current effective treatments and consider incorporating aspects of analytical therapy into their treatment of children with Asperger Syndrome if they deem it possibly beneficial to the child, using the therapy in conjunction with a multidisciplinary team.

Jungian Play Techniques with Autistic Children
Analysis and Interpretation

The aim of Jungian Play Therapy with autistic children is to provide a facilitative environment where psychological disturbances, which include the underpinnings of complex defenses, may be reached. However, analysis, which typically occurs four to five times per week, is not a financially realistic or logistical option for most families today. Therefore, the term *therapy,* as in Jungian Play Therapy, is more often utilized by this author to connate the less frequent (usually twice-per-week) therapeutic sessions. One of the inherent difficulties in using analytical play infrequently is the issue of working through resistances. Specifically, if children on the autism spectrum are seen infrequently, they may not sufficiently work through the effects of some of the interpretations because of the expanse of time between play sessions. They build resistances to the interpretations, possibly, to ward off anxieties (Fordham, 1976, 1994a). Moreover, the value of the play therapist's interpretations may become lost between sporadic sessions, thereby creating inherent difficulties when working through complexes.

I typically set appointments with children twice per week to meet the realistic demands of families' complicated schedules and still provide adequate support to the needs of the child's ego.

Furthermore, the analysis of children affected by autism encompasses toys and symbolic play for therapeutic purposes, yet the main component of child analysis is in the therapist's verbalizing and interpreting the action in the playroom and urging the child to do so as well (Allan, 1988; Fordham, 1976; Green, 2008, 2010a). Therefore, analytical play therapy would only be appropriate with sufficiently verbal, high-functioning children on the autism spectrum. The purpose of interpretation is to bring unconscious contents into awareness and to help the child mediate anxiety. The technique of interpretation does not relieve anxiety because the therapist tells the child something new about himself; rather, it gives the child information about her therapist's capacity to (a) hear her, (b) see her, (c) understand her, and (d) ultimately accept her. Interpretation is a key inductive technique when working with children with Asperger Syndrome as it (a) provides the child the abilities to resolve interpersonal deficiencies constellated in the transference and (b) relies on the use of symbols and the theory of archetypes to facilitate children's understanding of their fears and fantasies. Through interpretation, Jungian play therapists link symbolic play with personal observations and relevant experiences in the child's external world.

One last component of analysis and interpretation specific to working with children with Asperger Syndrome is the reliance on interpretation based upon the analyst's own counter-transference. Some children with Asperger Syndrome may find interpretations to be persecutory. If a child displays a manageable degree of persecutory tendencies during interpretation, this may be a sign that development is occurring. For example, I had a child client on the autism spectrum who continuously covered his ears when I provided verbalization of play. I gave a voice to the child's transference by stating, "You experience me as bad sometimes." Afterward, the child smiled and nodded his head. There was a sense of mutual understanding that had not occurred before this moment.

When there is repeated failure to get any type of response from a child with Asperger Syndrome during therapeutic interpretations (and the therapist hasn't been overly complicated with his language or ill-timed), the therapist should consider stopping and later conducting interpretation. This interpretation is not so much based inductively on the observable evidence in the child but more upon the therapist's own counter-transference. For example, I once had a 5-year-old client who did not want to leave the play session when it ended. The child charged into the waiting room area and began to harshly scream at and berate his mother, telling her he hated her and that he wished she would die. The mother's eyes began to well with tears. I felt distressed and realized that an interpretation based upon observable data may not have been effective. So I used his counter-transferential feelings and stated, "Now I feel like crying too because you're hurting your mother's feelings." The child instantly stopped his dysregulated behaviors, calmed himself down, then left without any other protestations. According to Fordham (1976), affective processes activated in the therapist through the counter-transference and sensitively verbalized to the child can be highly effective in promoting change in the child's behaviors.

Case Illustration

Joe, a child diagnosed with Asperger Syndrome, was 7 years old when I first met him in the playroom. He had been referred to me by his behavioral analyst. At that time, he was being treated by a multi-disciplinary team, including the behaviorist, who would visit him at school two times per week for 30 minutes, a school psychologist who had him partaking in group counseling and provided him psycho-education on Asperger Syndrome, and a pediatric neurologist. A comprehensive assessment for Asperger Syndrome was done a few months before I began counseling him, including a detailed developmental history and review of social, communication, and behavioral development. Specifically, his chart included data from psychometric assessments including the WISC-R and the Autism Diagnostic Observation Schedule, which was used to observe social behaviors at school necessary for a diagnosis. The Autism Diagnostic Observation Schedule is a semi-structured interview that requires established reliability and is conducted by clinicians who specialize in autism spectrum disorders; the interview includes free play (Toth & King, 2008). The results of Joe's assessments indicated a child who scored high in intelligence, had a low frustration tolerance, was socially inhibited, and scored exceptionally high in creativity and imaginative abilities. His history showed that he had intact cognitive ability (absence of mental retardation or intellectual disability) and no delays in early language milestones but was disproportionately anxious. His primary therapy was applied behavioral analysis, and he received social skills competency training from his school psychologist. His comprehensive treatment accentuated his strengths, targeted specific areas of impairment (socialization and academics) as well as comorbid medical or psychiatric disorders, and was implemented across settings to ensure success and generalization of skills. I was brought in as a targeted intervention specialist to augment his more broad-based intervention approaches to assist him in making meaningful connections with peers.

His mother informed me at our first interview that Joe needed help with identifying and expressing his feelings and improving his capacity to be comfortable in social situations with peers, especially during the school day. According to his chart and later corroborated by his mother and one of his teachers, there were many incidents at school in which teachers reported that Joe would withdraw and refuse to comply with directions and further learning. This seemed to be a product of a distressful social interaction Joe would have with peers. Fortunately, all of the adults I spoke to and observed interacting with Joe seemed fond of him and showed him care and respectful treatment. Joe was fully integrated into a private school in the southern portion of the United States. His grades fluctuated between straight A's, and periodic C's in science and reading. I conducted my own extended developmental assessment, including observing him at school, at home interacting with his family (composed of a mother, a father, and one younger brother), and in the playroom. I also conducted consultations with his teachers, his principal, and his close family members (including his grandparents on his mother's side), who provided input into Joe's current psychosocial struggles. The consensus was that Joe was benefiting from the behavioral analysis; he was learning to mediate his anxiety in school and at home. His mother was directly involved with the behavioral treatment and was open and receptive to feedback regarding changes in parenting and discipline to more fully support her son.

As for his presenting problems, some of the children at school were teasing him about being different because he was quiet and often introverted. His mother indicated that a couple of the boys at his school called him "weird." His mother reported that there were a couple of incidents at home in which he became intensely angry and violently threw things at her or tried to break whatever was in front of him. She remarked that these hostile occurrences were not frequent and were usually precipitated by her trying to comfort him after a difficult day at school. She also commented that one of his repetitive behaviors was staring at himself in front of the bathroom mirror for long periods of time in silence. She was advised by the behaviorist not to disrupt this activity unless it induced stress in the child.

I worked primarily with Joe's mother, since his father had a demanding work schedule and was often unavailable for consultations. She and I met every two weeks for a parent consultation. Joe's parents were both highly educated and would be classified in the upper middle class socioeconomically. They had tremendous resources and utilized their financial leverage to assist their child by securing services. Joe had a primarily positive relationship with both of his parents. He would draw things for them and regularly sit next to either one while watching TV in the living room. They also provided him and his brother lots of positive attention and were seemingly content. There was no indication or admission of trauma, neglect, or abuse in Joe's childhood history. Joe also had a significant social support system with his extended family members, who would visit the household multiple times a month. I worked with Joe twice per week for approximately five months.

IMPLEMENTATION OF JUNGIAN PLAY THERAPY MODEL

During our first two weeks of play therapy, Joe was relatively quiet. He regularly engaged in symbolic and spontaneous play, especially gravitating toward the sand tray and the figurines. He spent most of our time together during this initial, *orientation* phase massaging the sand with his hands and creating chaotic sand worlds in silence. When I attempted to discuss the sand scenes with him afterward, he did not respond to my questions. He validated my initial clinical impression that he lived primarily in an interior world. Also, he would color mandalas and would not finish them but rather give up before they were completed (fig. 9.1).

I began using interpretations as he built the sand pictures after the first couple of weeks, and then, interestingly, he began to verbalize. The first verbal communication involved his sand world of chaos and destruction. It was filled with little green army men and one red dragon and one green dragon with fire coming out of its mouth. The dragons would annihilate all of the army men, and Joe would make death-cry sounds as the army men perished. I made the interpretation, "Seems like the dragons are really angry at the army men and want to show them how powerful they are." I interpreted that he was projecting his inner world of splitting between good and bad objects, possibly similar to what he experienced day after day at school as he

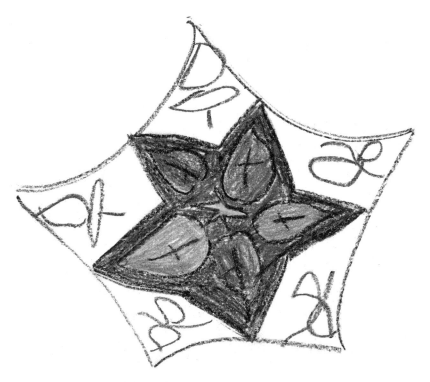

Figure 9.1. Joe's mandala no. 1

wanted to be accepted by peers but did not know how to connect. Therefore, he split and saw others as bad and needing to be destroyed (children sometimes use the death or *thanatos* wish to convey disappearance or removal of things or people). His play began to modify slightly after I began making interpretations while he created his sand worlds of destructive violence and carnage. At one point, he made a laughing noise with the red dragon after he knocked several dead army men out of the sand tray. I responded, "He's happy now that those army men won't hurt him any longer. He's showing them that he's not going to be hurt anymore." Joe's anxious play began to diminish, and for the first time, he responded, "Yes, the dragon hates these bad guys because they're trying to kill him, and he just wants to live." I analyzed this interaction as Joe differentiating between good and bad self-objects that were being projected into the sand scene. On the one hand, he was feeling omnipotent because he was closely identifying with the symbol of the dragon, who was breathing fire. Jung referred to creating fire as an instinctive behavior related to rhythmic activities from a primitive source. I interpreted Joe's use of fire to destroy the army men as part of his psyche's *prima materia* being activated in the symbolic play constellation. This provided me with an inference about his unconscious affect, whether defensive or instinctual, that needed to be explored further.

During the next couple of months, Joe's play could be primarily characterized as the *working-through* phase. He began verbalizing more. He added tremendous narrative content to his sand worlds and seemed to have developed a sense of trust in the analytical relationship. I would make interpretations during his play, and he would sometimes respond and other times continue playing as if he hadn't heard me. As time passed on, some of his sand worlds become anxious and aggressive. I permitted this intense display of aggression because I wanted to uncover the core of his hostility. I needed to ascertain the ideas, fantasies, and beliefs connected with this rage. Some of his violent play included throwing some of the army men at the wall and replying, "Now you're dead bitch!" I would not stop his affective display of rage, but interpreted, "I bet sometimes you wish some of those mean boys at your school would disappear so they can't hurt you anymore." At this point, I interpreted that he was living in a terrorized state. His projections consistently depicted his experience of fantastic ideas and objects as inherently maligning. He exteriorized his conflicts, and I made reflective statements to show him I understood how scary his inner world could be at times. After hearing this comment, he responded acutely, "Yes, they don't like me and I don't know why." His aggression began to sublimate into sadness or despair at this point. It is these feelings that are so important for the therapist to discriminate, because these underlying feelings, which prompt a child's rage, are more important than the rage itself. In this moment, Joe reached out and began to internalize a good enough father imago within me. I replied, "It sounds like you want to be liked and accepted but don't know how to make friends and that makes you feel different and strange."

After hearing this last interpretation, he began to cry. He came over to where I was sitting and gave me a hug. This was the first time in our six weeks or so of therapy up to that point that Joe physically acknowledged my presence. Before, I was simply another object in the playroom. And he sat there, for a couple of minutes, and cried. I comforted him, and then he sat on a chair across from me and looked down at the floor. I remember his mother telling me that she would offer advice to her son about making friends and sometimes became frustrated when Joe wouldn't follow her instruction, which would prompt his raging at home. Instead of trying to rescue the child from his despair (which I believe he was anticipating that I would do), I let him sit with the pain. Jung said to get through the depression, we must enter it. And that was an extremely difficult moment for me to get through as a clinician; I was experiencing counter-transference of wanting to protect him and shield him from the psychogenic pain he was experiencing. The session ended with grounding the child back to his external reality. I asked him to color a mandala. He created an intricate design with dark hues of colors, including black, deep red, and brown. The mandala he chose was complex in that it contained multiple shapes and was shaded with intense, bold, dark hues of colors (fig. 9.2). This activity seemed to noticeably calm his affect. Research has found that coloring mandalas can be a soothing activity that decreases anxiety (Henderson, Rosen, Mascaro, 2007). When the session ended, he gave me a hug and said "Goodbye."

During next several weeks of therapy, Joe remained limited in his verbal interactions with me. His mother began reporting he appeared less anxious at home and had no meltdowns, and his teachers found him to be less obstinate in class. It seems as though he was indeed aware of his feelings but not overly concerned or even aware of the feelings of others. Sometimes it seemed as though I was doing therapy alone; he seemed emotionally detached from the play. As the therapy continued, Joe began to manipulate a small mirror sand figurine. At first, he would include it in his sand scenes by placing it impulsively in the world without much discernible reason. Then he began making it the centerpiece of his play. His mother disclosed to me during our interviews that Joe would sometimes stare in the mirror at home for long periods of time. I interpreted his scenes, but I could get no response. His mind was expressing its aptitude for symbolic expression, but I had not yet recognized the myth in which his psyche was unfolding.

During our sessions, I would sometimes read fairy tales or myths to him and ask him to sand a world afterward. During one session, I read the Greek myth of Echo and Narcissus. I explained to him how a mountain nymph (and love-struck admirer) named Echo chased after the beautiful god boy Narcissus, who was not all that interested in her. Narcissus had been pursued by many maidens but was excessively proud and wanted nothing to do with them. Echo could use her voice only to repeat back the last few words of the other person during a conversation. One day, she attempted to pro-

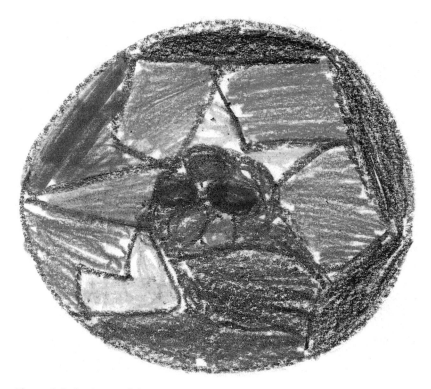

Figure 9.2. Joe's mandala no. 2

fess her love for Narcissus in the forest, and proud Narcissus coldly rejected her. He thought she was a lowly handmaiden, and he wanted nothing to do with her and her repetitive words. One day Narcissus went out hunting and stopped at a fountain to drink. He saw a beautiful image, his reflection. Not knowing it was his him, he admired the reflection. He became enamored by it, so much that he stayed at that fountain staring and talking to his own image. Narcissus withered and turned into a flower after realizing that the image in the fountain was a reflection, like a mirror, and therefore incapable of expressing love. He died lonely and heartbroken. I asked Joe to sand a picture from the story. He made an immediate comparison as he was smoothing the sand, "Me and him both like mirrors." I replied, "Yes, it seems as though you two have something in common."

Joe then sanded a picture with a small blue pool in the middle of the tray. Next to the pool was one male figure and one princess fairy figurine, and a mirror was placed in between the two figures. I asked him to tell me about the scene. "Echo wants to get close to Narcissus. But he doesn't like her because she bothers him. So he told her to leave him alone. But she won't. So he put a mirror between them so she couldn't see him, and he could see himself. He liked looking at himself because it was better than looking at Echo." In this projective scene, I interpreted Joe connecting to the elements inherent within the myth and correlating his subjective experience of feeling socially isolated and alone. Because he did not have the capacity to form social bonds, perhaps it was easier for him and less anxiety-provoking for him to isolate himself behind a facade or mirror. I responded, "What would happen if Narcissus removed the mirror?" Joe hesitantly looked at me, and responded emphatically, "He wouldn't!" So I tried again, "I'm wondering what it would be like if Narcissus felt that Echo wouldn't hurt him. Maybe if he trusted others and himself more? What would it be like then?" Joe stood quietly for a moment, then removed the mirror between them and placed it to the side. He said, "Narcissus would probably talk to her and tell her he just wants people to like him." So I instructed him to talk through the characters and tell me what it would sound like. He went on to describe Narcissus and Echo having a conversation about taking turns swimming in the pool, but Narcissus told Echo she couldn't ever stare at him too long. Shortly after this scene ended, I asked Joe to draw a mandala before he left. In his mandala, he depicted a large circle with a blue star in the middle. He also placed some blue star stickers on the mandala. I asked him what the title of his mandala was, and he responded with a smile, "me."

During our next session, he continued sanding a picture with Narcissus and Echo until the mirror finally disappeared and Echo and Narcissus were seemingly friends. He said they enjoyed playing together. I made the interpretation, "Joe, seems like Narcissus finally let his guard down. Even after being bothered by other nymphs, he finally allowed himself to get close to Echo, and she was nice to him. And he realized he could make friends with Echo and maybe other nymphs if he just trusted in himself. Removing that mirror was a big, scary step." He slightly accepted my interpretation, saying, "Yeah, maybe so." Shortly after this session, the mother reported to me that Joe asked if he could have a play date with another boy at his school. This was the first play date Joe had ever been on, surprisingly. She asked if I had suggestions to make things go OK so he would want to do it again, and I responded, "Trust yourself and him and let him be who he is. He needs to play and figure out who he is in relation to others. If things don't go well, he'll figure out how to improve. Or maybe he'll ask your help." That play date went well, fortunately. The mother said the boys played with Joe's Star Wars Lego set and built a scene, and there was no tension.

The following week (*the reparation/termination stage*), Joe spent most of our playtime sanding a world with a castle and many fairies at the top of a mountain he built with moon sand. He placed a gold jewel at the bottom of the mountain. I asked him to tell me about the story of his scene. He said that the fairy princesses had finally found their lost golden egg. One of the princesses had dropped it when she was playing, but they found it and now everyone is happy because it's magical. The psychology of the child archetype here, mainly the "divine child," was activated. Joe identified in this symbolic play with an omnipotent power that was regained and brought great joy to everyone in the kingdom. He produced the symbols, and he followed them through carnage and war to magic golden eggs. At this point in therapy, I knew we had gone as far as we could go. Joe was showing small increments of improvement in his attitude at school and was starting to make new friends. His play had transformed from scattered, chaotic, violent, to organized, coherent, and even mystical. Also, his mandalas reflected cooler, less intense colors, and he depicted a calming sense of content from his narratives related to the image (fig. 9.3).

During this time, he began building trust with others because some of the children who were teasing him stopped. The school psychologist and I worked together to formulate a guidance curriculum on bullying. It seems to have alleviated some of the harassment he and other children were experiencing. Also, though still quiet and seemingly comfortable with being alone, Joe started to try to apply his own unique style of relating to objects to people. As he had worked through conflicts in the sand world, he began to externalize his newfound inner reserves. He began to trust in himself and realize that he was worthy to make friends with others, and that they wouldn't always hurt him.

POST-ANALYSIS

Joe's outcome within the Jungian play psychotherapy trajectory was relatively positive. My goals were to enhance his ego-Self axis so that he had a strong, valid connection between his rich inner world and his sometimes bewildering outer world. Second, I wanted to help him develop a symbolic attitude so that he would follow symbols and allow them to lead to healing.

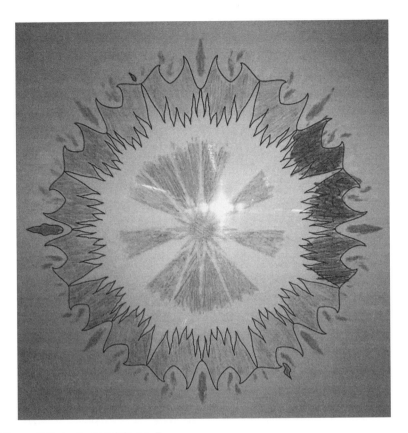

Figure 9.3. Joe's mandala no. 3

Also, we aimed to help him feel more comfortable with making social bonds. Before this occurred, Joe needed to internalize that he could trust others and they would not always hurt him. Though Joe's myth-making may have looked like pure archetypal imagery, there were clear links between his inner and outer realities. He was able to see his *potential future,* as Jung described it (Fordham, 1976), inherent within the symbolic expressions of the self-symbols related to the Narcissus myth. This identification helped compensate his conscious attitude with instinctual root systems of belief, including the potential for wholeness. Once he saw that Narcissus was not happy being alone with only his reflection, he was able to make the affective shift in his own self-alienation. I hypothesized that Joe's individuating function had already been set in motion before he began working with me, based upon his material. His strong family and school support systems were working hard to create a cohesive environment for this child. Though I believe some of my interpretations were facilitative, there is clear evidence that this child was on his own path to growth. The dialectic was never severed for too long, which undoubtedly helped Joe, as our biweekly sessions provided a holding effect for his anxieties surrounding socialization. After analyzing this case, I have come to realize that my analysis and playtime with him was subsidiary: I did not cure him of his social woes but only provided an environment in which his own therapy was nurtured.

Conclusion

The clinician looking to incorporate analytical play with a child with Asperger Syndrome should do so only in the context of sufficient training with symbol work and in conjunction with a multi-disciplinary team of professionals. Furthermore, the clinician will want to have a solid foundation in sandplay and the archetypal imagery inherent throughout. Second, clinicians should be advised that interpretations are extremely important when facilitating change by using analytical play. Therefore, only highly verbal and high-functioning children with autism would be appropriate with this modality. Last, clinicians need to know beforehand that it can at times be a lonely place in the playroom, since a hallmark of this population is the difficulty to socially or empathically connect with others. Therefore, clinicians wanting to work with this population by using analytical play should approach it with care and collaborative reliance upon the support of other professionals in the field. By reaching out to the inner dimensions of a child with Asperger Syndrome with compassion and dynamic understanding, clinicians are able to help children mitigate psychological obstacles so that they may see their own resplendent reflections, out of which meaningful social bonds may be formulated.

Integrative Jungian Play Therapy

Synthesizing Trauma, Transformation,

and Transcendence

Every one of us carries a deforming mirror where he sees himself too small or too large or too fat or too thin. Once the deforming mirror is smashed, there is the possibility of wholeness, there is the possibility of joy.

—Anaïs Nin

———

This brief concluding chapter provides the culminating synthesis of the content areas presented in this book: integrative Jungian Play Therapy with children that ultimately synthesizes trauma, transformation, and transcendence.

According to Drewes (2012), the integration of theoretical rationale, clinical process, and theory—specific interventions in child psychotherapy—has proliferated among practicing clinicians. Once referred to as *eclecticism, integrative therapy* is the common term used now to describe the synthesis of theory and skill to best meet a client's needs from a holistic perspective. Traditionally, *eclectic* within the psychotherapeutic context equated to clinicians selecting different theories and interventions as a prescriptive approach to meet clients where they are developmentally. However, Drewes (2012) discusses how to transform the kitchen-sink approach of eclecticism into a more academically refined "integration," whereby various theories are applied to one interactive and coordinated means of treatment.

Schaefer (2003) (as cited in Drewes, 2012) stated that because children's psychopathology is often multi-layered, complex, and multi-determined from familial influences, a multi-modal treatment approach is required.

Play therapists trained in one theoretical paradigm, including those trained within the analytical framework, concur that their singular theory of choice and training often does not fully capture the complexities of a modern human soul. Drewes (2012) goes on to comment that there is little to no empirical evidence demonstrating that one approach (i.e., Gestalt, Solution-Focused, Psychoanalytic) exacts psychotherapeutic change for all psychological disorders and the dynamic patients that display them. Integrative play therapy theories incorporate a blending of various aspects of the client's personal experience in the present "here and now" moment. This incorporation or integration highlights the importance of the therapeutic feedback loop as well as the byproduct of containment of raw material presented and/or activated within the consulting room by the patient (Drewes, 2012). To competently apply this ultimate synthesis of theory and skill with diverse clients in real situations, play therapists adhere to an integrative approach in treatment with children. They do not, as previously seen as a norm in the psychotherapeutic community, stoically or defiantly hold on to one theory without adapting or changing, based upon a misplaced loyalty. In addition, subtle behavioral changes over time from participation in the play therapy process and relationship can potentially lead to broad reverberations and changes throughout all aspects of the client's maladaptive functioning (Drewes, 2012).

The current and comprehensive research being done in mental health treatment with traumatized children has resulted in "evidence-based practices" that advocate for an integrative treatment approach that involves expressive arts, play, and the features of cognitive behavioral paradigms that target disordered behaviors (Drewes, 2012). Thus, expressive arts, play, and developmentally appropriate creative activities have been found to be beneficial and necessary when assisting children in integrating their traumatic experiences in meaningful ways, such as embracing transcendence (van der Kolk & d'Andrea, 2010).

Currently, cognitive behavioral therapy (CBT), an empirical-based approach, is demonstrated as "effective" and decreases many of the negative symptoms associated with childhood trauma. Jungian Play Therapy is a potentially beneficial intervention that (a) is developmentally sensitive to self-modulating hyper-arousal, (b) facilitates emotional safety by utilizing less threatening forms of communication such as symbols and metaphors rather than the standard "talking cure," (c) engenders attention to inner processes that are often resisted by those affected by trauma, (d) fosters self-efficacy in collaborative problem solving, and (e) promotes trust through a non-judgmental, therapeutic relationship. The play therapist's development and nurturing of an empathic therapeutic relationship with the child, alongside integrating play with trauma treatment protocols that remain sensitive to the internal processes, may facilitate a "sacred space" (or *temenos*) that assists with successful trauma transformation into integration and hopefully transcendence.

Integrating Jungian Play Therapy with Evidence-Informed Interventions

While there are numerous interventions tailored for child and adolescent trauma treatment, much of the evidence-based research focuses on CBT. CBT has been consistently demonstrated as effective in reducing post-traumatic stress, decreasing feelings of dysphoria or depression, and diminishing hyper-arousal. The theoretical assumption of CBT is that an adolescent's faulty perceptions of a traumatic event lead the adolescent to structure thoughts into rigid, maladaptive beliefs and behavioral patterns. Trauma triggers (or reminders) in the adolescent's environment may further intensify negative reactions or feelings. Recognizing and restructuring these cognitive distortions is a critical goal in CBT work with traumatized children.

For some children and adolescents, writing about aberrant thoughts and feelings surrounding a traumatic experience and then depicting them symbolically through play-based media like sandplay and abstract artwork is less threatening than expressing the information verbally and may assist with trauma integration. Prominent trauma researchers van der Kolk and d'Andrea (2010) state that simply talking about traumatic experiences does not necessarily assist the mind and brain to integrate the dissociated images and cognitions into a cohesive whole. As in most CBT therapies, the therapeutic dyad between the play therapist and the child is critical for healing. Through play-based therapy sessions, child patients and their play therapists engage in co-participating activities that further the child's trust in others and increase the opportunities for post-traumatic integration to occur. A Jungian play-based integration materializes when play therapists incorporate sandplay or drawings to assist children in focusing attention on their internal experience while introducing cognitive, affective, and sensorimotor elements of their trauma. Jungian play-based media to assist children in paying closer attention to their internal sensations and perceptions may include (a) a sand tray and sand miniatures with which children create pictures in the sand and share glimpses of their internal state symbolically, (b) the use of acrylic art with canvases on an easel to produce abstract imagery and symbols within diverse cultural and sociological contexts; and (c) individually constructed multicolored sand mandalas or predrawn mandalas to color on paper using pencils and markers.

Integrating Jungian Play Therapy and Trauma-Focused Cognitive Behavioral Therapy

Trauma-focused cognitive behavioral therapy (TF-CBT) is a variation of CBT in that it is specific to children and adolescents who have experienced traumatic events and have sustained substantial psychological deficits. TF-CBT is based upon six core values. The first is that it is component based, meaning it has a collection of core skills that assist and build upon one another. Second is the value of respect: respect for the individual, as well as family's religious, community, and cultural values. The third core value is adaptability. It is the play therapist's primary responsibility to be flexible and creative when selecting which components of TF-CBT will be utilized with children or adolescents. The fourth core value is family involvement. The fifth core value is the therapeutic relationship; play therapists model trust, empathy, and acceptance throughout the treatment process. The final value is the instillment of self-efficacy. In any therapy, ideal functioning is typically instilled within the client during, and most importantly, after treatment. The common curative factor in many of these therapeutic interventions is the play therapist's commitment to fostering resiliency and promoting wellness. This is achieved partially by ensuring that adolescents experience self-mastery of trauma exposure and are able to autonomously modulate their arousal states. Additionally, the integration of Jungian play-based interventions, such as when a play therapist leads a child in guided imagery and the child then colors a mandala and writes out the story of the mandala from an internal perspective, further provides opportunities to increase self-awareness in the present moment. Van der Kolk and d'Andrea (2010) comment that effective therapy specific to resolving childhood interpersonal trauma increases the individual's physical self-experience and self-awareness, as opposed to remaining fixated on making meaning of the trauma narrative of the past.

Resilience and Jungian Play-Based Techniques: Integrative Approaches

Resilience is the ability to adapt and utilize effective coping skills in the face of adversity, trauma, tragedy, threats, or even significant sources of distress. The National Child Traumatic Stress Network lists four core components in fostering resiliency. The number one factor in resiliency is feeling safe in one's environment. Children who do not feel psychosocially safe at school are less likely to develop the supportive relationships that help them thrive. Play therapists are in a position to provide the opportunity for healthy socialization and encourage critical reflection on maintaining personal safety and security. Another resiliency component is "traumatic experiences integration," which includes "meaning-making," "traumatic memory containment," and "mourning traumatic loss." Next is "relational engagement," where strong adult attachments are essential. The last core component is "positive affect enhancement," focusing on positive self-esteem and achievement by mastering play or activity-based board games, competitive yet fantastical video games, and cooperative activities (Green, 2012a, 2012b).

Jungian Play Therapy may be integrated into resiliency practices to augment the healing trajectory for traumatized children. Specifically, the use of cooperative board games played by play therapists and children (or perhaps the play therapist listens to lyrics of popular songs the child brings into the session related to socialization or self-expression) and the honoring and containing of the symbols associated with these activities helps children internalize stable social connections, explore opportunities for self-discovery, and nurture a positive, more realistic view of the self. Personal characteristics that promote trauma integration and foster resiliency (which a play therapist can model through puppet shows or simple role plays) include (a) an easygoing disposition, (b) a positive temperament, (c) an analytical attitude that honors and follows symbols, and (d) the cultivation of special talents, creativity, and spirituality.

Integrative Jungian Play Therapy: Conclusion

Incorporating a Jungian play-based modality alongside an evidence-based treatment protocol may facilitate a salubrious environment that promotes trauma transformation into a meaningful integration and personal transcendence (Green, 2012a, 2012b). The use of manualized, highly structured, and/or clinically rigid "evidence-based" treatment protocols requires the flexibility and warmth of a play therapist to see traumatized children as unique individuals in their own right and not simply diagnostic labels to be cured or fixed. Integrative Jungian Play Therapy, including the person-centered or humanistic therapeutic dyad as the centerpiece, alongside the ability to use directive techniques such as coloring mandalas and resolving trauma narratives symbolically in sandplay, while combating or disputing irrational beliefs to formulate a more accurate cognitive appraisal, may benefit children's successful integration of trauma. Jungian play therapists must receive training in research-based and trauma treatment protocols, including TF-CBT, as well as being open and receptive to clinical supervision, when integrating play. Even though much of the research in treating trauma focuses on CBT, Jungian Play Therapy and generic play-based interventions are listed as "not ineffective" and may assist children in the exploration and successful resolving of stress related to traumatic events. The therapeutic relationship remains the most salient curative factor throughout the treatment process, because it allows the play therapist to model trust, empathy, and unconditional acceptance. And symbols produced by the child are seen as valid forms of communication to be amplified within the consulting room, where containment may occur. During and after the process of a successful integration of trauma, children begin to believe in their ability to prevail beyond adversity. And eventually their faith in others may become restored as well, as they see the world, once again, as safe, stable, and secure. Finally they may again imagine the future without desolation. They see a "positive potential future," which is not filled with harm, but one where they feel OK about themselves and the world around them.

Final Reflection

Now that you've completed the journey of reading this book and finding your own path toward integrating Jungian Play Therapy into your practice, let's close with a final activity. Just as the mandala is circular, we shall end where we began. Complete another sand picture or mandala. Afterward, reflect. Now, go back and look at your first creations from when you begin this journey. What differences do you notice? What similarities? How have you grown? How have your given depth a voice within your own soul? What final reflection do you have about your own growth and personal attainment? After you're done reflecting, quiet your mind. Submerge in complete silence for 15 minutes or longer. Breathe. An answer will come to you. That answer is for you and you only. It is the numinous message from the soul. You've now reconnected to your archetypal imagination. Go out and play. Use play dough. Read a novel. Pick petals off a flower. Giggle. Watch a cartoon. Eat cookie dough. And know that you are always enough. Your creativity, alone, will decide. And I wish you light and love as you journey on, dedicating your career to helping the most vulnerable among us—our children. There is no finer calling.

Appendix
Specialized Training: Becoming a Sandplay Therapist

Selected Books and DVDs on Sandplay
Sandplay: A Psychotherapeutic Approach to the Psyche, by Dora M. Kalff
Sandplay: Past, Present, and Future, by Harriet S. Friedman and Rie Rogers Mitchell
Sandplay: Silent Workshop of the Psyche, by Kay Bradway and Barbara McCoard
*Sandplay and Storytelling: The Impact of Imaginative Thinking on Children's Learning and
    Development*, by Barbara A. Turner and Kristin Unnsteinsdottir
Supervision of Sandplay Therapy, by Harriet S. Friedman and Rie Rogers Mitchell

Selected Books on Integrating Play Therapy and Sandplay with Children
Handbook of Jungian Play Therapy, by Eric J. Green
Inscapes of the Child's World, by John Allan
Sandplay: Therapy with Children and Families, by Lois J. Carey
Sandplay Therapy in Vulnerable Communities: A Jungian Approach, by Eva Zoja

Selected Sandplay Therapy DVDs
Jungian Play Therapy and Sandplay with Children, by Eric J. Green (Alexander Street Press)
Sandplay: What It Is and How It Works, by Gita Morena (Sandplay Video Productions)

Helpful Links
The Sandplay Therapists of America: www.sandplay.org/links.htm
Colorado Sandplay Therapy Association: Research & Training Institute:
    www.sandplaytherapy.org
Center for Jungian Studies of South Florida: www.jungcentersouthflorida.org
International Society for Sandplay Therapy: www.isst-society.com
Canada: The Canadian Association of Sandplay Therapists: www.sandplay.ca
Israel: The Israeli Sandplay Therapist Association: www.sandplay.co.il

Select Sandplay Trainings in the United States
Dee Preston-Dillon: http://sandplayvoices.blogspot.com
Rosalind L. Heiko: www.drheiko.com/training/sandplay-training-heiko
Sandplay Therapists of America Annual Conference: www.sandplay.org/training
    _conferences.htm#Conferences

References

Aldwin, C. M. (1994). *Stress, coping, and development: An integrative perspective.* New York: Guilford Press.

Allan, J. (1988). *Inscapes of the child's world: Jungian counseling in schools and clinics.* Dallas, TX: Spring.

Allan, J. (1997). Jungian play psychotherapy. In K. J. O'Connor & L. M. Braverman (eds.), *Play therapy: A comparative presentation* (pp. 100–130). New York: John Wiley.

Allan, J., & Berry, P. (1987). Sandplay. *Elementary School Guidance and Counseling,* 24:300–306.

Allan, J., & Bertoia, J. (1992). *Written paths to healing: Education and Jungian child counseling.* Dallas, TX: Spring.

Allan, J., & Brown, K. (1993). Jungian play therapy in elementary schools. *Elementary School Guidance and Counseling,* 28:5–25.

Allan, J., & Clark, M. (1984). Directed art counseling. *Elementary School Guidance and Counseling,* 19:116–24.

Allen, J. P., & Land, D. (1999). Attachment in adolescence. In J. Cassidy & P. R. Shaver (eds.), *Handbook of attachment: Theory, research, and clinical applications* (pp. 319–35). New York: Guilford Press.

American Psychiatric Association (APA). (2000). *Diagnostic and statistical manual of mental disorders.* 4th ed., text rev. Arlington, VA: Author.

Anderson, R. A. (1993). As the child plays, so grows the family tree: Family play therapy. In T. Kottman & C. E. Schaefer (eds.), *Play therapy in action: A casebook for practitioners* (pp. 457–83). Northvale, NJ: Jason Aronson.

Association for Play Therapy. (2012). *Play therapy clinical definition.* Retrieved April 5, 2012, from www.a4pt.org/ps.index.cfm?ID=2289.

Ayyash-Abdo, H. (2001). Childhood bereavement: What school psychologists need to know. *School Psychology International,* 22:417–33.

Baggerly, J. N., & Green, E. J. (2013). Playing in peril after a natural disaster: Incorporating play therapy with responsive services. In J. Curry & L. Fazio-Griffith (eds.), *Integrating play techniques in comprehensive school counseling programs* (pp. 149–65). New York: Information Age.

Baggerly, J., Ray, D., & Bratton, S. (eds.) (2010). *Child-centered play therapy research: The evidence base for effective practice.* Hoboken, NJ: John Wiley.

Bailey, C. E. (ed.) (2000). *Children in therapy: Using the family as a resource.* New York: W. W. Norton.

Bailey, C. E., & Sori, C. F. (2000). Involving parents in children's therapy. In Bailey, 2000 (pp. 475–501).

Barnitz, L. (2001). Effectively responding to the commercial sexual exploitation of children: A comprehensive approach to prevention, protection, and reintegration services. *Child Welfare,* 80:597–610.

Barth, J. C. (2006). Families coping with the death of a parent: The therapist's role. In L. Combrinck-Graham (ed.), *Children in family contexts: Perspectives on treatment* (pp. 312–30). New York: Guilford Press.

Batts, J. (2004). Death and grief in the family: Providing support at school. In A. S. Canter, L. Z. Paige, M. D. Roth, I. Romero, & S. A. Carroll (eds.), *Helping children at home and school II: Handouts for families and educators* (pp. S9-S15). Bethesda, MD: National Association of School Psychologists.

Beaucaire, M. (2012). *The art of mandala meditation.* Avon, MA: Adams Media (division of F+W Media).

Becker-Blease, K. A., Turner, H. A., & Finkelhor, D. (2010), Disasters, victimization, and children's mental health. *Child Development,* 81:1040–52.

Benz, U., & Axelrod, T. (2004). Traumatization through separation: Loss of family and home as childhood catastrophes. *Shofar,* 23 (1): 85–99.

Berger, L. E., Jodl, K. M., Allen, J. P., McElhaney, K. B., & Kuperminc, G. P. (2005). When adolescents disagree with others about their symptoms: Differences in attachment organization as an explanation of discrepancies between adolescent, parent, and peer reports of behavior problems. *Development and Psychopathology,* 17:509–28.

Berlin, L. J., & Cassidy, J. (1999). Relations among relationships: Contributions from attachment theory and research. In J. Cassidy & P. R. Shaver (eds.), *Handbook of attachment: Theory, research, and clinical applications* (pp. 688–712). New York: Guilford Press.

Bertrone, A., Mottrron, L., Jelenic, P., & Faubert, J. (2005). Enhanced and diminished visuo-spatial information processing in autism depends on stimulus activity. *Brain,* 128 (10): 2430–41.

Black, D. S., Grenard, J. L., Sussman, S., & Rohrbach, L. A. (2010). The influence of school-based natural mentoring relationships on school attachment and subsequent adolescent risk behaviors. *Health Education Research,* 25:892–902.

Black, S. (2001). Disaster's aftermath. *American School Board Journal,* 4:188.

Boik, B. L., & Goodwin, E. A. (2000). *Sandplay therapy.* New York: W. W. Norton.

Bonny, H., & Kellogg, J. (1977). Mandalas as a measure of change in psychotherapy. *American Journal of Art Therapy,* 16:126–30.

Botkin, D. (2000). Family play therapy: A creative approach to including young children in family therapy. *Journal of Systemic Therapies,* 19 (3): 31–42.

Bowlby, J. (1960). Grief and mourning in infancy and early childhood. *Psychoanalytic Study of the Child,* 15:99–112.

Bowlby, J. (1982). *Attachment and loss.* 2nd ed. New York: Basic.

Bradway, K., & McCoard, B. (2005). *Sandplay: Silent workshop of the psyche.* New York: Routledge.

Bratton, S. C., Ray, D., Rhine, T., & Jones, L. (2005). The efficacy of play therapy with children: A meta-analytic review of treatment outcomes. *Professional Psychology,* 36:376–90.

Briere, J., & Elliot, D. M. (2003). Prevalence and symptomatic sequelae of self-reported childhood physical and sexual abuse in a general population sample of men and women. *Child Abuse and Neglect,* 27:1205–22.

Briere, J., & Scott, C. (2006). *Principles of trauma therapy: A guide to symptoms, evaluations, and treatment.* Thousand Oaks, CA: Sage.

Briggs, S. (2003). *Working with adolescents: A contemporary psychodynamic perspective.* New York: Palgrave Macmillan.

Bryan, T., Burstein, K., & Ergul, C. (2004). The social-emotional side of learning disabilities. A science-based presentation of the state of the art. *Learning Disability Quarterly,* 27:45–51.

Brymer, M., Jacobs, A., Layne, C., et al. (2006). *Psychological first aid: Field operations guide.* 2nd ed. National Child Traumatic Stress Network and National Center for PTSD. Available at www.nctsn.org.

Buchalter, S. (2013). *Mandala symbolism and techniques: Innovative approaches for professionals.* Philadelphia: Jessica Kingsley.

Buist, K. L., Dekovic, M., Meeus, W., & van Aken, M. A. G. (2004). The reciprocal relationship between early adolescent attachment and internalizing and externalizing problem behavior. *Journal of Adolescence,* 27:251–66.

Busch, T., & Kimble, C. S. (2001). Grieving children: Are we meeting the challenge? *Pediatric Nursing,* 27:414–18.

Buschgens, C. J. M., van Aken, M. A. G., Swinkels, S. H. N., et al. (2008). Differential family and peer environmental factors are related to severity and comorbidity in children with ADHD. *Journal of Neural Transmission,* 115:177–86. Retrieved March 29, 2008, from Academic Search Premiere database.

Campbell, J. (2008). *The mythic dimensions: Selected essays, 1959–1987.* Novato, CA: New World Library.

Carey, L. (1990). Sandplay therapy with a troubled child. *The Arts in Psychotherapy,* 17:197–209.

Carey, L. (1991). Family sandplay therapy. *The Arts in Psychotherapy,* 18:231–39.

Carey, L. (1994). Family sandplay therapy. In Schaefer & Carey, 1994 (pp. 205–19).

Carey, L. (1999). *Sandplay therapy with children and families.* Northvale, NJ: Jason Aronson.

Carey, L. (2006a) *Expressive and creative arts methods for trauma survivors.* London: Jessica Kingsley.

Carey, L. (2006b). Short-term family sandplay therapy. In H. Kaduson & C. E. Schaefer (eds.), *Short-term play therapy for children* (pp. 202–15). New York: Guilford Press.

Caron, M. J., Mottron, L., Rainville, C., & Chouinard, S. (2004). Do high functioning persons with autism present superior spatial abilities? *Neurospsychologia,* 42 (4): 467–81.

Carroll, J. (1995). Non-directive play therapy with bereaved children. In S. C. Smith & M. Pennells (eds.), *Interventions with bereaved children* (pp. 68–83). Bristol, PA: Jessica Kingsley.

Castro-Blanco, D., & Karver, M. S. (eds.) (2010). *Elusive alliance: Treatment engagement strategies with high-risk adolescents.* Washington, DC: American Psychological Association.

Chodorow, J. (2006). Active imagination. In R. Papadopoulos (ed.), *The handbook of Jungian psychology* (pp. 215–43). London: Routledge.

Chorpita, B. F., Becker K. D., Daleiden, E. L. (2007). Understanding the common elements of evidence-based practice: Misconceptions and clinical examples. *Journal of American Academic Child and Adolescent Psychiatry, 46*:647–52.

Cohen, J. A., Mannarino, A. P., & Deblinger, E. (2006). *Treating trauma and traumatic grief in children and adolescents.* New York: Guilford Press.

Couch, J. B. (1997). Behind the veil: Mandala drawings by dementia patients. *Art Therapy, 14* (3): 187–93.

Cox, C. T., & Cohen, B. M. (2000). Mandala artwork by clients with DID: Clinical observations based on two theoretical models. *Art Therapy, 17*:195–201.

Crenshaw, D. A. (2005). Clinical tools to facilitate treatment of childhood traumatic grief. *OMEGA, 51*:239–55.

Crenshaw, D. A. (2008). Multiple sources of child wounding and paths to healing. In D. A. Crenshaw (ed.), *Child and adolescent psychotherapy: Wounded spirits and healing paths* (pp. 1–14). Lanham, MD: Jason Aronson.

Curry, N. A., & Kasser, T. (2005). Can coloring mandalas reduce anxiety? *Journal of the American Art Therapy Association, 22*:81–85.

Deblinger, E., Behl, L. E., & Glickman, A. R. (2006). Treating children who have experienced sexual abuse. In P. Kendall (ed.), *Child and adolescent therapy: Cognitive behavioral strategies* (pp. 177–99). New York: Guilford Press.

Deblinger, E., & Runyon, M. E. (2005). Understanding and treating feelings of shame in children who have experienced maltreatment. *Child Maltreatment, 10*:364–76.

DeCosse, D. E. (2007). Freedom of the press and Catholic social thought: Reflection on the sexual abuse scandal in the Catholic church in the United States. *Theological Studies, 68*:865–99.

De Domenico, G. (1994). Jungian play therapy techniques. In K. J. O'Connor & C. E. Schaefer (eds.), *Handbook of play therapy: Advances and innovations* (pp. 253–82). 2nd ed. New York: John Wiley.

Dermer, S., Olund, D., & Sori, C. F. (2006). Integrating play in family therapy theories. In C. F. Sori (ed.), *Engaging children in family therapy: Creative approaches to integrating theory and research in clinical practice* (pp. 37–65). New York: Routledge.

Doka, K. J. (ed.) (2000). *Living with grief: Children, adolescents, and loss.* Philadelphia: Brunner-Mazel.

Donald, B. (2003). Self-regulation in the repair of an adolescent boy's early insecure attachment. *Journal of Sandplay Therapy, 12* (1): 109–30.

Drewes, A. (ed.) (2009). *Blending play therapy with cognitive behavioral therapy: Evidence-based and other effective treatments and techniques.* Hoboken, NJ: John Wiley.

Drewes, A. (2012). Integrative play therapy. In A. Drewes, S. Bratton, & C. Schaefer (eds.), *Integrative play therapy* (pp. 21–36). Hoboken, NJ: Wiley.

Duchesne, S., & Larose, S. (2007). Adolescent attachment to mother and father and academic motivation and performance in early adolescence. *Journal of Applied Social Psychology, 37*:1501–21.

Dunne, E. (2004). Clerical child sex abuse: The response of the Roman Catholic Church. *Journal of Community and Applied Social Psychology*, 14:490–94.

Eliot, A. O. (2009). Adolescent alliance building: A contemporary approach to an ancient concept. *Annals of the American Psychotherapy Association*, 12 (3): 10–16.

Fincher, S. (2000). *Coloring mandalas 1: For insight healing and self-expression.* Boston: Shambhala.

Fincher, S. (2009). *The mandala workbook. A creative guide for self-exploration, balance, and well-being.* Boston, MA: Shambhala.

Finkelhor, D., & Berliner, L. (1995). Research on the treatment of sexually abused children: A review and recommendations. *Journal of the American Academy of Child and Adolescent Psychiatry*, 34:1408–23.

Fiorini, J. J., & Mullen, J. A. (2006). *Counseling children and adolescents through grief and loss.* Champaign, IL: Research Press.

Fordham, M. (1976). *The self and autism.* London: William Heinemann Medical Books.

Fordman, M. (1988). Emergence of child analysis. In Sidoli & Davies, 1988 (pp. 19–29).

Fordham, M. (1994a). *Children as individuals.* London: Free Association Books.

Fordham, M. (1994b). *The life of childhood.* London: Routledge.

Fox, G. (2006). Development in family contexts. In L. Combrinck-Graham (ed.), *Children in family contexts: Perspectives on treatment* (pp. 26–50). New York: Guilford Press.

Froehlich, T. E., Lanphear, B. P., Epstein, J. N., Barbaresi, W. J., Katusic, S. K., Kahn, R. S. (2007). Prevalence, recognition, and treatment of attention-deficit/hyperactivity disorder in a national sample of US Children. *Archives of Pediatric and Adolescent Medicine*, 16 (9): 857–64.

Fry, V. L. (2000). Part of me died too: Creative strategies for grieving children and adolescents. In Doka, 2000 (pp. 125–37).

Furman, W., Simon, V. A., Shaffer, L., & Bouchey, H. A. (2002). Adolescents' working models and styles for relationships with parents, friends, and romantic partners. *Child Development*, 73:241–55.

Furman, W., & Wehner, E. A. (1997). Adolescent romantic relationships: A developmental perspective. *New Directions for Child Development*, 78:21–36.

Furth, G. M. (1988). *The secret world of drawings: Healing through art.* Boston, MA: SIGO Press.

Gaffner, D. C., & Hazler, R. J. (2002). Factors related to indecisiveness and career indecision in undecided college students. *Journal of College Student Development*, 43:317–26.

Gaines, J. (2006). Law enforcement reactions to sex offender registration and community notification. *Police Practice and Research*, 7:249–67.

Gil, E. (1994). *Play in family therapy.* New York: Guilford Press.

Gil, E. (2003). Family play therapy: "The bear with short nails." In C. E. Schafer (ed.), *Foundations of play therapy* (pp. 192–218). Hoboken, NJ: John Wiley.

Gil, E. (2006). *Helping abused and traumatized children: Integrating directive and nondirective approaches.* New York: Guilford Press.

Gil, E. (2011). *Helping abused and traumatized children: Integrating directive and nondirective approaches.* New York: Guilford Press.

Gil, E., & Sobol, B. (2000). Engaging families in therapeutic play. In Bailey, 2000 (pp. 341–82).

Glazer, H. R., & Clark, M. D. (1999). A family-centered intervention for grieving preschool children. *Journal of Child and Adolescent Group Therapy*, 9 (4): 161–68.

Goldman, L. (2001). *Breaking the silence: A guide to help children with complicated grief.* 2nd ed. New York: Brunner-Routledge.

Goodheart, W. (1980). Review of Langs' and Searles' books. *San Francisco Jung Institute Library Journal*, 1 (4): 2–39.

Gordon, R. (1993). *Bridges: Metaphor for psychic processes.* London: Karnac.

Graetz, B., Sawyer, M., Baghurst, P., & Hirte, C. (2006). Gender comparisons of service use among youth with attention-deficit/hyperactivity disorder. *Journal of Emotional and Behavioral Disorders*, 14 (1): 2–11. Retrieved Feb. 17, 2008, from Academic Search Premier database.

Grandin, T. (2006). *Thinking in pictures: My life with autism.* 2nd ed. New York: Vintage Books.

Green, E. (2004). Activating the self-healing archetype: Spontaneous drawings with children affected by sexual abuse. *Association for Play Therapy Newsletter*, 23 (4): 19–20.

Green, E. (2005). Jungian play therapy: Bridging the theoretical to the practical. *VISTAS: Compelling Perspectives on Counseling*, 1:75–78.

Green, E. J. (2006). Jungian play therapy: Activating the self-healing archetype in children affected by sexual abuse. *Louisiana Journal of Counseling*, 8:1–11.

Green, E. (2007). The crisis of family separation following traumatic mass destruction: Jungian analytical play therapy in the aftermath of hurricane Katrina. In N. B. Webb (ed.), *Play therapy with children in crisis: Individual, group, and family treatment* (pp. 368–88). 3rd ed. New York: Guilford Press.

Green, E. J. (2008). Re-envisioning Jungian analytical play therapy with child sexual assault survivors. *International Journal of Play Therapy*, 17 (2): 102–21.

Green, E. J. (2009a). Jungian analytical play therapy. In K. J. O'Connor & L. D. Braverman (eds.), *Play therapy theory and practice: Comparing theories and techniques* (pp. 83–122). 2nd ed. Hoboken, NJ: John Wiley.

Green, E. J. (2009b). Teaching self-empowerment skills gives children a voice. *ASCA School Counselor*, 13 (3): 11–17.

Green, E. J. (2010a). Jungian play therapy with adolescents. *Play Therapy*, 5 (2): 20–23.

Green, E. J. (2010b). Traversing the heroic journey: Jungian play therapy with children. *Counseling Today*, 52 (9): 40–43.

Green, E. J. (2012a). Facilitating resiliency in traumatized adolescents: Integrating play therapy with evidence-based interventions. *Play Therapy*, 6 (3): 10–15.

Green, E. J. (2012b). The Narcissus myth, resplendent reflections, and self-healing: A contemporary Jungian perspective on counseling high-functioning Autistic children. In L. Gallo-Lopez, & L. Rubin (eds.), *Play based interventions for children and adolescents with autism spectrum disorders* (pp. 177–92). London: Routledge.

Green, E. J. (2013). *Mandalas and meaning: A coloring workbook for adolescents.* Dallas, TX: Author.

Green, E., & Christensen, T. (2006). Children's perceptions of play therapy in school settings. *International Journal of Play Therapy*, 15(1): 65–85.

Green, E. J., & Connolly, M. (2009). Jungian family sandplay with bereaved children: Implications for play therapists. *International Journal of Play Therapy*, 18 (2): 84–98.

Green, E. J., Crenshaw, D., & Kolos, A. (2010). Counseling children with preverbal trauma. *International Journal of Play Therapy, 19*(2): 95–105.

Green, E. J., Crenshaw, D., & Langtiw, C. (2009). Play theme-based research with children. *Family Journal, 17*(4): 312–17.

Green, E. J., & Drewes, A. (eds.) (2013). *Integrating expressive arts with play therapy: A guidebook for mental health practitioners and educators.* Hoboken, NJ: John Wiley.

Green, E. J., Drewes, A. & Kominski, J. (2013). The use of mandalas in Jungian play therapy with adolescents diagnosed with ADHD: Implications for play therapists. *International Journal of Play Therapy, 22* (3): 159–72.

Green, E. J., & Gibbs, K. (2010). Jungian sandplay for preschool children with disruptive behavioral problems. In C. Schaefer (ed.), *Play therapy for preschool children* (pp. 223–44). Washington, DC: American Psychological Association.

Green, E., & Hebert, B. (2006). Serial drawings: A Jungian play therapy technique for caregivers to utilize with children between counseling sessions. *Play Therapy, 1* (4): 20–24.

Green, E. J., & Ironside, D. (2004). Archetypes, symbols, and Jungian sandplay: An innovative approach to school counseling. *Counselor's Classroom.* Retrieved Sept. 22, 2007, from www.guidancechannel.com.

Green, E. J., Myrick, A., & Crenshaw, D. (2013). Toward secure attachment in adolescent relational development: Advancements from sandplay and expressive play-based interventions. *International Journal of Play Therapy, 22* (2): 90–102.

Green, E. J., Schweiker, K., Kolos, A., & Keith, K. (2009). *Empirical-based play techniques with resistant adolescents.* Research proposal presented at a symposium for the American Counseling Association Annual World Conference, Charlotte, NC.

Gren-Landell, M., Tillfors, M., Furmark, T., Bohlin, G., Andersson, G., & Svedin, C. (2009). Social phobia in Swedish adolescents: Prevalence and gender. *Social Psychiatry and Psychiatric Epidemiology, 44*:1–7.

Hahm, H. C., Lahiff, M., & Guterman, N. B. (2003). Acculturation and parental attachment in Asian-American adolescents' alcohol use. *Journal of Adolescent Health, 33*:119–29.

Hay, I., & Ashman, A. F. (2003). The development of adolescents' emotional stability and general self-concept: The interplay of parents, peers, and gender. *International Journal of Disability, Development, and Education, 50*:77–91.

Hebert, B., & Green, E. (2005, April). Activation of the self-healing archetype: Counseling children affected by sexual abuse within a Jungian context. Paper presented at the American Counseling Association World Conference, Atlanta, GA.

Heflin, A. H., & Deblinger, E. (2007). Child sexual abuse. In F. M. Dattilio & A. Freeman (eds.), *Cognitive-behavioral strategies in crisis intervention* (pp. 247–76). 3rd ed. New York: Guilford Press.

Henderson, A. J. Z., Bartholomew, K., Trinke, S. J., & Kwong, M. J. (2005). When loving means hurting: An exploration of attachment and intimate abuse in a community sample. *Journal of Family Violence, 20* (4): 219–30.

Henderson, P. G. (2007). Creativity, expression, and healing: An empirical study using mandalas within the written disclosure paradigm. Master's thesis, Texas A&M University. Retrieved Feb. 5, 2013, from http://repository.tamu.edu/bitstream/handle/1969.1/ETD-TAMU-1604/HENDERSON-THESIS.pdf.

Henderson, P., Rosen, D., & Mascaro, N. (2007). Empirical study on the healing nature of mandalas. *Psychology of Aesthetics, Creativity, and the Arts,* (1) 3: 148–54.

Hetzel-Riggin, M. D., Brausch, A. M., & Montgomery, B. S. (2007). A meta-analytic investigation of therapy modality outcomes for sexually abused children and adolescents: An exploratory study. *Child Abuse and Neglect,* 31:126–41.

Homeyer, L. E., & Sweeney, D. S. (2005). Sandtray therapy. In C. A. Malchiodi (ed.), *Expressive therapies* (pp. 162–82). New York: Guilford Press.

Howard, M. S., & Medway, F. J. (2004). Adolescents' attachments and coping with stress. *Psychology in the Schools,* 41:391–402.

Hunter, S. V. (2006). Understanding the complexity of child sexual abuse: A review of the literature with implications for family play therapists. *Family Journal,* 14:349–58.

Jaycox, L. H., Cohen, J. A., Mannarino, A. P., et al. (2010). Children's mental health care following Hurricane Katrina: A field trial of trauma-focused psychotherapies. *Journal of Traumatic Stress,* 23 (2): 223–31.

Jung, C. G. (1910). *Psychic conflicts in the child.* In H. Read, M. Fordham, & G. Adler (eds.), *The collected works of C. G. Jung,* vol. 17. Princeton, NJ: Princeton University Press.

Jung, C. G. (1913). *The theory of psychoanalysis.* In H. Read, M. Fordham, & G. Adler (eds.), *The collected works of C. G. Jung,* vol. 4. Princeton, NJ: Princeton University Press.

Jung, C. G. (1951). The psychology of the child archetype. In H. Read, M. Fordham, & G. Adler (eds.), *The collected works of C. G. Jung,* vol. 9. Princeton, NJ: Princeton University Press.

Jung, C. G. (1959). *Collected works 9: The archetypes and the collective unconscious.* New York: Pantheon.

Jung, C. G. (1963). *Memories, dreams, and reflections.* New York: Pantheon.

Jung, C. G. (1964). *Man and his symbols.* Garden City, NY: Doubleday.

Jung, C. G. (1973). *Mandala symbolism.* Trans. R. F. C. Hull. Bollingen Series. Princeton, NJ: Princeton University Press.

Jung, C. G. (2008). *Children's dreams: Notes from the seminar given in 1936–1940.* Princeton, NJ: Princeton University Press.

Jung, C. G. (2009). *The red book.* New York: W. W. Norton.

Kalff, D. (1980). *Sandplay: A psychotherapeutic approach to the psyche.* Boston: Sigo Press.

Kalsched, D. (1996). *The inner world of trauma: Archetypal defenses of the personal spirit.* New York: Routledge.

Kavale, K. A., Holdnack, J. A., & Mostert, M. P. (2005). Social skills interventions for individuals with learning disabilities. *Learning Disabilities Quarterly,* 27:31–45.

Kellogg, J., Mac Rae, M., Bonny, H. L., & di Leo, F. (1977). The use of the mandala in psychological evaluation and treatment. *American Journal of Art Therapy,* 16 (4): 123–34.

Kestley, T. (2010). Group sandplay in elementary schools. In A. Drewes & C. Schaefer (eds.), *School-based play therapy* (pp. 257–82). 2nd ed. Hoboken, NJ: John Wiley.

Klein, M. (ed.) (1955). *New directions in psycho-analysis.* New York: Basic Books.

Knell, S., & Dasari, M. (2009). CBPT: Implementing and integrating CBT into clinical practice. In Drewes, 2009 (pp. 321–52).

Kronenberg, M. E., Hansel, T., Brennan, A. M., Osofsky, H. J., Osofsky, J. D., & Lawrason, B. (2010). Children of Katrina: Lessons learned about postdisaster symptoms and recovery patterns. *Child Development,* 81 (4): 1241–59.

La Greca, A. (2008). Interventions for posttraumatic stress in children and adolescents following natural disasters and acts of terrorism. In R. C. Steele, T. D. Elkin, & M. C. Roberts (eds.), *Handbook of evidence-based therapies for children and adolescents: Bridging science and practice* (pp. 121–41). New York: Springer Science.

La Greca, A. M., & Silverman, W. K. (2009). Treatment and prevention of posttraumatic stress reactions in children and adolescents exposed to disasters and terrorism: What is the evidence? *Child Development Perspectives,* 3 (1): 4–10.

Landreth, G. (2001). *Innovations in play therapy: Issues, process, and special populations.* Philadelphia: Brunner-Routledge.

Landreth, G. L. (2002). *Play therapy: The art of the relationship.* 2nd ed. New York: Brunner-Routledge.

Landreth, G. L. (2012). *Play therapy: The art of the relationship.* 3rd ed. New York: Brunner-Routledge.

Landreth, G. L., Baggerly, J., & Tyndall, A. L. (1999). Beyond adapting adult counseling skills for use with children: The paradigm shift to child-centered play therapy. *Journal of Individual Psychology,* 55 (3): 272–88.

Larose, S., & Boivin, M. (1998). Attachment to parents, social support expectations, and socioemotional adjustment during the high school–college transition. *Journal of Research on Adolescence,* 8 (1): 1–27.

LeBlanc, M., and Ritchie, M. (1999). Predictors of play therapy outcomes. *International Journal of Play Therapy,* 8 (2): 19–34.

Levenson, J. S., D'Amora, D. A., & Hern, A. L. (2007). Megan's law and its impact on community re-entry for sex offenders. *Behavioral Sciences and the Law,* 25:587–602.

Lilly, J. P. (2009). Jungian analytical play therapy: Theory and practice. Proposal presented at the Annual Association for Play Therapy International Conference, Atlanta, GA.

Liu, Y. (2007). Paternal/maternal attachment, peer support, social expectations of peer interaction, and depressive symptoms. *Adolescence,* 41:705–21.

Liu, Y. (2008). An examination of three models of the relationships between parental attachments and adolescents' social functioning and depressive symptoms. *Journal of Youth and Adolescence,* 37:941–52.

Liu, M., Shih, W., & Ma, L. (2011). Are children with Asperger syndrome creative in divergent thinking and feeling? A brief report. *Research in Autism Spectrum Disorders,* 5 (1): 294–98.

Lowenfeld, M. (1979). *The world technique.* Boston: Allen & Unwin.

Lu, L., Petersen, F., Lacroix, L., & Rousseau, C. (2010). Stimulating creative play in children with autism through sandplay. *The Arts in Psychotherapy,* 37 (1): 56–64.

Lund, L. K., Zimmerman, T. S., & Haddock, S. A. (2002). The theory, structure, and techniques for the inclusion of children in family therapy: A literature review. *Journal of Marital and Family Therapy,* 28:445–54.

Maddocks, A., Griffiths, L., & Antao, V. (1999). Detecting child sexual abuse in general practice: A retrospective case-control study from Wales. *Scandinavian Journal of Primary Health Care,* 17:210–14.

Mahar, D. J., Iwasiw, C. L., & Evans, M. K. (2012). The mandala: First-year undergraduate nursing students' learning experiences. *International Journal of Nursing Education Scholarship,* 9 (1): 23–35.

Main, M., & Solomon, J. (1990). Disordered attachment. In M. Greenberg, D. Cicchetti, &

M. Cummings (eds.), *Attachment in the preschool years: Theory, research, and intervention* (pp. 121–60). Chicago: University of Chicago Press.

Main, S. (2008). *Childhood re-imagined*. New York: Routledge.

Marcum, C. D. (2007). Interpreting the intentions of Internet predators: An examination of online predator behaviors. *Journal of Child Sexual Abuse,* 16:99–114.

Marshall, W. L. (1997). Pedophilia: Psychopathology and theory. In D. R. Laws & W. O'Donohue (eds.), *Sexual deviance: Theory, assessment, and treatment* (pp. 152–74). New York: Guilford Press.

Mauk, G. W., & Sharpnack, J. D. (2006). Grief. In G. G. Bear & K. M. Minke (eds.), *Children's needs III: Development, prevention, and intervention* (pp. 239–54). Bethesda, MD: National Association of School Psychologists.

Maxwell, L. A., & Holovach, R. (2007). Digital age adds new incidents to staff-student sex. *Education Weekly,* 27:1–14.

McGee, R., Williams, S., Howden-Chapman, P., Martin, J., & Kawachi, I. (2006). Participation in clubs and groups from childhood to adolescence and its effects on attachment and self-esteem. *Journal of Adolescence,* 29:1–17.

McNulty, W. (2007). Superheroes and sandplay: Using the archetype through the healing journey. In L. C. Rubin (ed.), *Using superheroes in counseling and play therapy* (pp. 69–89). New York: Springer.

Melvin, D., & Lukeman, D. (2000). Bereavement: A framework for those working with children. *Clinical Child Psychology and Psychiatry,* 5:521–39.

Miller, M. A. (1995). Re-grief as a narrative: The impact of parental death on child and adolescent development. In D. W. Adams & E. J. Deveau (eds.), *Helping children and adolescents cope with death and bereavement* (pp. 99–113). Amityville, NY: Baywood.

Mitchell, R. R., Friedman, H. & Green, E. J. (2014). Integrating play therapy and sandplay therapy. In E. Green & A. Drewes (eds.), *Integrating expressive arts and play therapy with children and adolescents* (pp. 101–24). Hoboken, NJ: John Wiley.

Moody, R. A., & Moody, C. P. (1991). A family perspective: Helping children acknowledge and express grief following the death of a parent. *Death Studies,* 15:587–602.

Moore, T. (2008). *A life at work: The joy of discovering what you were born to do.* New York: Broadway Books.

Multon, K. D., Heppner, M. J., Gysbers, N. C., Xook, C. E., & Ellis-Kalton, C. (2001). Client psychological distress: An important factor in career counseling. *Career Development Quarterly,* 49:324–35.

Muris, P., Meesters, C., Morren, M., & Moorman, L. (2004). Anger and hostility in adolescents: Relationships with self-reported attachment style and perceived parenting rearing styles. *Journal of Psychosomatic Research,* 57:257–64.

National Child Traumatic Stress Network. (2012). Response to natural disasters. Retrieved April 5, 2012, from www.nctsn.org/trauma-types/natural-disasters/tornadoes#tabset-tab-5.

Nomaguchi, K. M. (2008). Gender, family structure, and adolescents' primary confidants. *Journal of Marriage and Family,* 70:1213–27.

Oaklander, V. (1978). *Windows to our children.* Moab, UT: Real People Press.

Oltjenbruns, K. A. (2001). Developmental context of childhood: Grief and regrief phenomena. In M. S. Stroebe, R. O. Hansson, W. Stroebe, & H. Schut (eds.), *Handbook of bereavement research: Consequences, coping, and care* (pp. 169–97). Washington, DC: American Psychological Association.

Orcutt, H. K., Garcia, M., & Pickett, S. M. (2005). Female-perpetrated intimate partner violence and romantic attachment style in a college student. *Violence and Victims,* 20:287–302.

Pane, J., McCaffrey, D. F., Kalra, N., & Zhou, A. (2008). Effects of student displacement in Louisiana during the first academic year after the hurricanes of 2005. *Journal of Education for Children Placed at Risk,* 13 (2): 168–211. Available at www.rand.org/pubs /reprints/2008/RAND_RP1379.pdf.

Patton, J. (2006, Aug.). Jungian spirituality: A developmental context for later-life growth. *American Journal of Hospice and Palliative Medicine,* 23 (4): 304–8. Retrieved Jan. 5, 2008, from PsycINFO database.

Pearson, M., & Wilson, H. (2001). *Sandplay and symbol work: Emotional healing and personal development with children, adolescents, and adults.* Melbourne, Victoria: Australian Council for Educational Research.

Peery, J. C. (2003). Jungian analytical play therapy. In C. E. Schaefer (ed.), *Foundations of play therapy* (pp. 14–54). Hoboken, NJ: John Wiley.

Perl, E. (2008). *Psychotherapy with adolescent girls and young women: Fostering autonomy through attachment.* New York: Guilford Press.

Piaget, J. (1962). *Play, dreams, and imitation in childhood.* New York: Routledge.

Pizarro, J. (2004). The efficacy of art and writing therapy: Increasing positive mental health outcomes and participant retention after exposure to traumatic experience. *Art Therapy,* 21 (1): 5–12.

Polt, N. (2005). Coloring mandalas with adults in a short-term inpatient psychiatric hospital. Master's thesis, Ursuline College. Retrieved Jan. 18, 2013, from Proquest Digital Dissertations database.

Preston-Dillon, D. (2007). *Sand therapy: An introduction.* Audio course. Fresno, CA: Association for Play Therapy.

Putnam, F. W. (2003). Ten-year research update review: Child sexual abuse. *Journal of the American Academy of Child and Adolescent Psychiatry,* 42:269–78.

Raffaelli, M., Crockett, L. J., & Shen, Y. L. (2005). Developmental stability and change in self-regulation from childhood to adolescence. *Journal of Genetic Psychology,* 166 (1): 54–76.

Rasmussen, L. A., & Cunningham, C. (1995). Focused play therapy and non-directive play therapy: Can they be integrated? *Journal of Child Sexual Abuse,* 4:1–20.

Reddy, L. A., Files-Hall, T. M., & Schaefer, C. E. (2005). Announcing empirically based play interventions for children. In L. A. Reddy, T. M. Files-Hall, & C. E. Schaefer (eds.), *Empirically based play interventions for children* (pp. 3–10). Washington, DC: American Psychological Association.

Reyes, J. P. M., Shirk, S. R., Labouliere, C. D., & Karver, M. (2010). Adolescent alliance: Predictor or outcome? Paper presented at the American Psychological Association Convention, San Diego, CA.

Rosenfeld, L. B., Caye, J. S., Ayalon, O., & Lahad, M. (2005). *When their world falls apart: Helping families and children manage the effects of disasters.* Washington, DC: NASW Press.

Rosenn, D. (2009). Asperger connections 2008 keynote speech. *Asperger's Association of New England Journal,* 4:5–8.

Rotter, J. C., & Bush, M. V. (2000). Play and family therapy. *Family Journal*, 8:172–76.

Rowe, E., & Eckenrode, J. (1999). The timing of academic difficulties among maltreated and nonmaltreated children. *Child Abuse and Neglect*, 23:813–32.

Saarikallio, S., & Erkkilä, J. (2007). The role of music in adolescents' mood regulation. *Psychology of Music*, 35 (1): 88–109.

Samuels, A. (2006). Transference/countertransference. In R. Papadopoulos (ed.), *The handbook of Jungian psychology* (pp. 177–95). London: Routledge.

Schaefer, C. E. (2003). Prescriptive play therapy. In C. E. Schaefer (ed.), *Foundations of Play Therapy* (pp. 306–20). Hoboken, NJ: Wiley.

Schaefer, C., & Carey, L. (eds.) (1994). *Family play therapy*. Northvale, NJ: Jason Aronson.

Schultz, P. D. (2005). *Not monsters: Analyzing the stories of child molesters*. Lanham, MD: Rowman & Littlefield.

Sedgwick, D. (2001). *Introduction to Jungian psychotherapy: The therapeutic relationship*. New York: Taylor & Francis.

Seiffge-Krenke, I. (2006). Coping with relationship stressors: The impact of different working models of attachment and links to adaptation. *Journal of Youth and Adolescence*, 35:25–39.

Seligman, E. 2006. *The half-alive ones: Clinical papers on analytical psychology in a changing world*. London: Karnac.

Shapiro, E. A. (1994). *Grief as a family process: A developmental approach to clinical practice*. New York: Guilford Press.

Shelby, J. S. (2007). *Everything you want to know about child sexual assault survivors: From forensics to treatment*. Handout. Hollywood, CA: Author.

Shelby, J. S., & Felix, E. D. (2005). Posttraumatic play therapy: The need for an integrated model of directive and nondirective approaches. In L. A. Reddy, T. M. Files-Hall, & C. E. Schaefer (eds.), *Empirically based play interventions for children* (pp. 79–104). Washington, DC: American Psychological Association.

Shelton, K. H., & van den Bree, M. B. M. (2010). The moderating effects of pubertal timing on the longitudinal associations between parent-child relationship quality and adolescent substance abuse. *Journal of Research on Adolescence*, 20:1044–64.

Shen, Y. J. (2002.) Short-term group play therapy with Chinese earthquake victims: Effects on anxiety, depression, and adjustment. *International Journal of Play Therapy*, 11 (1): 43–63.

Sherwood, D. N. (2007). The traditional Plains Indian vision quest: Initiation and individuation. In E. Kirsch, V. B. Rutter, & T. Singer (eds.), *Initiation: The living reality of an archetype* (pp. 103–22). New York: Routledge.

Shih, Y. L., Kao, S. S., & Wang, W. H. (2006). The process study of the sandplay therapy on oppositional defiant disorder. *Chinese Annual Report of Guidance and Counseling*, 19:41–72.

Shunsen, C. (2010). The principles and operations of sandplay therapy on children with autism. *Chinese Journal of Special Education*, 4 (3): 011–022.

Sidoli, M., & Davies, M. (eds.) (1988). *Jungian child psychotherapy: Individuation in childhood*. London: Karnac Books.

Silverman, P. R. (2000). *Never too young to know: Death in children's lives*. New York: Oxford University Press.

Simons, K. J., Paternite, C. E., & Shore, C. (2001). Quality of parent/adolescent attachment and aggression in young adolescents. *Journal of Early Adolescence,* 21:182–203.

Slegelis, M. H. (1987). A study of Jung's mandala and its relationship to art psychotherapy. *The Arts in Psychotherapy,* 14:301–11.

Smitherman-Brown, V., & Church, R. P. (1996). Mandala drawing: Facilitating creative growth in children with ADD or ADHD. *Art Therapy,* 13:252–62.

Speece, M. W., & Brent, S. B. (1996). The development of children's understanding of death. In C. A. Corr & D. M. Corr (eds.), *Handbook of childhood death and bereavement* (pp. 29–50). New York: Springer.

Stein. R. (2007). Initiation as surrender: A twelve-year analysis. In E. Kirsch, V. B. Rutter, & T. Singer (eds.), *Initiation: The living reality of an archetype* (pp. 63–81). New York: Routledge.

Steinberg, L. (2007). Risk taking in adolescence: New perspectives from brain and behavioral science. *Current Directions in Psychological Science,* 16 (2): 55–59.

Steinhardt, L. (2000). *Foundation and form in Jungian sandplay.* Philadelphia: Jessica Kingsley.

Stevens, A. (2006, March 3). Sex-assault out *Women's eNews.* Retrieved April 16, 206, from www.womensenews.org/article.cfm?aid=2657.

Stroebe, W., & Schut, H. (2001). Risk factors in bereavement outcome: A methodological and empirical review. In M. S. Stroebe, R. O. Hansson, W. Stroebe, & H. Schut (eds.), *Handbook of bereavement research: Consequences, coping, and care* (pp. 349–71). Washington, DC: American Psychological Association.

Toth, K., & King, B. H. (2008). Asperger's syndrome: Diagnosis and treatment. *American Journal of Psychiatry,* 165:958–63.

Turner, B. A. (2005). *The handbook of sandplay therapy.* Cloverdale, CA: Temenos Press.

U.S. Department of Health & Human Services, Administration of Children, Youth, & Families. (2006). *Child maltreatment.* Washington, DC: U.S. Government Printing Office.

Van der Kolk, B., & d'Andrea, W. (2010). Towards a developmental trauma disorder diagnosis for childhood interpersonal trauma. In R. A. Lanius, E. Vermetten, & C. Pain (eds.), *Impact of early life trauma on health and disease* (pp. 57–68). Cambridge: Cambridge University Press.

Van Der Vennet, R., & Serice, S. (2013). Can coloring mandalas reduce anxiety? A replication study. *Art Therapy,* 29 (2): 97–92.

Van der Vorst, H., Engels, R. E., Meeus, W., Devokic, M., & Vermulst, A. (2006). Parental attachment, parental control, and early development of alcohol use: A longitudinal study. *Psychology of Addictive Behaviors,* 20:107–16.

Van Doorn, M. D., Branje, S. J. T., & Meeus, W. H. J. (2011). Developmental changes in conflict resolution styles in parent-adolescent relationships: A four-wave longitudinal study. *Journal of Youth and Adolescence,* 40:97–107.

Vignoli, E., Croity-Belz, S., Chapeland, V., de Fillipis, A., & Garcia, M. (2005). Career exploration in adolescents: The role of anxiety, attachment, and parenting style. *Journal of Vocational Behavior,* 67:153–68.

Walsh, D., & Allan, J. (1994). Jungian art counseling with the suicidal child. *Guidance and Counseling,* 10 (1): 3–10.

Way, P., & Bremner, I. (2005). Therapeutic interventions. In B. Monroe & F. Kraus (eds.), *Brief interventions with bereaved children* (pp. 65–80). New York: Oxford University Press.

Webb, N. B. (2000). Play therapy to help bereaved children. In Doka, 2000 (pp. 139–52).

Webb, N. B. (ed.) (2002). *Helping bereaved children: A handbook for practitioners.* New York: Guilford Press.

Webb, N. B. (2003). Play and expressive therapies to help bereaved children: Individual, family, and group treatment. *Smith College Studies in Social Work,* 73 (3): 405–22.

Webster, R. E. (2001). Symptoms and long-term outcomes for children who have been sexually assaulted. *Psychology in the Schools,* 38:533–47.

Widom, C. S. (1999). Posttraumatic stress disorder in abused and neglected children grown up. *American Journal of Orthopsychiatry,* 56:1223–29.

Winnicott, D. (1971). *Playing and reality.* New York: Basic Books.

Wolfe, B. S., & Senta, L. M. (1995). Interventions with bereaved children nine to thirteen years of age: From a medical center–based young person's grief support program. In D. W. Adams & E. J. Deveau (eds.), *Helping children and adolescents cope with death and bereavement* (pp. 203–27). Amityville, NY: Baywood.

Yalom, I. D. (1995). *The theory and practice of group psychotherapy.* New York: Basic Books.

Zylowska, L., Ackerman, D. L., Yang, M. H., et al. (2008). Mindfulness meditation training in adults and adolescents with ADHD. A feasibility study. *Journal of Attention Disorders,* 11:737–46.

Index

Page numbers in italics signify illustrations.